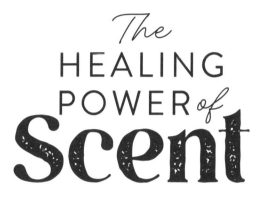

The HEALING POWER of Scent

DAVID & CHARLES

www.davidandcharles.com

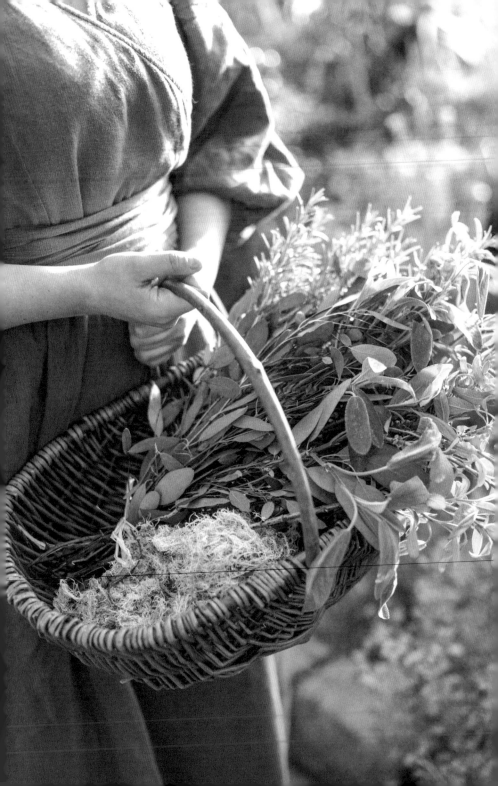

Contents

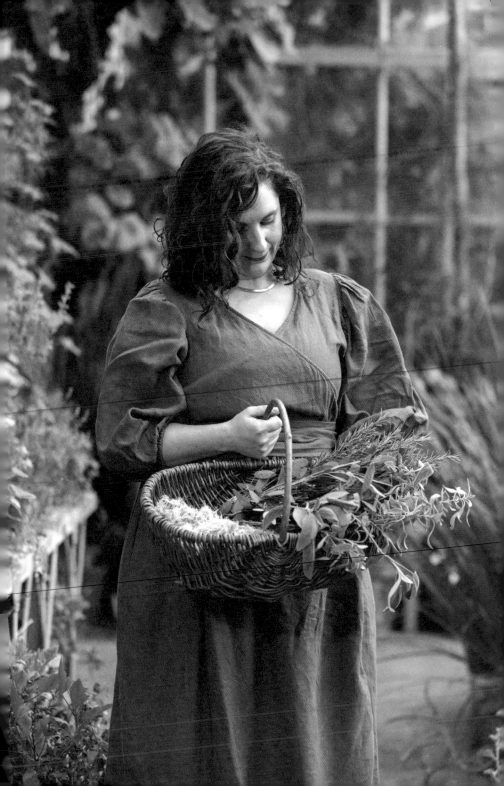

INTRODUCTION

My Journey with Scent

Scent	scent, n.
/sɛnt/	An odour or aroma; a distinctive or characteristic smell; esp. one that is pleasant.
	scent, v.
	To fill or imbue with a (usually pleasant) odour; to impart a smell to; to perfume.[1]

" Herbs and aromatherapy have provided a discreet, supportive backdrop throughout my life: I haven't always noticed them, but they have always been there, supporting me through the highs and lows of life. "

I spent my early career and most of my twenties hopping around in a series of supposedly meaningful yet ultimately unfulfilling roles, and moving house every year. Some of my workplaces were highly toxic, some were full of inspiring scientists and activists, and in some I even met a number of close friends. I worked in communications, marketing and business development across the international development, environmental and public health sectors – fascinating areas in themselves, and I wholly acknowledge my privilege in being able to say that I have worked in some world-recognised institutions. But as I moved from city to city, flatshare to flatshare, job to job, I kept hearing the voice at the back of my mind that said 'this isn't really who you are'. I know I've certainly seen a similar tale or two in the books I read whilst trying to figure out how to support my mental health better, find my community, and do something that I find meaningful with my life.

Perhaps unsurprisingly, as time went on, I suffered a series of existential mental health crises with long bouts of anxiety, panic and depression against the backdrop of ever-changing homes and jobs. I say this in full acknowledgement of the fortunate position I was in to have a supportive community of family members and friends alongside a doctor, herbalist and therapist, all of whom helped to pull me out of the woods – just enough for me to see that I needed to make some serious changes in my life.

Some years prior I had volunteered at a community herbal medicine centre in a Guatemalan river village, which had left me deeply changed. Since returning to the UK, I had not stopped thinking about my time there, learning about herbs, how accessible and intrinsic they had been to ancient Mayan life, and how important they still were to the health of communities on the Rio Dulce. I learned how necessary it was to preserve medicinal plant knowledge for the good of all. Indeed, at the time I visited, the community was so far from the nearest well-equipped hospital, and healthcare was so underfunded that having centres that promoted plant knowledge was all but essential.

Back to 2017, sitting on the floor in a South London flat, I didn't know exactly where I was heading, but I knew that my path lay in supporting others with their mental wellbeing, and working with plants in some way. Now in my mid-thirties, I have been diagnosed with ADHD, and I feel that this neurodivergent way of seeing and operating in the world was likely one of the reasons I felt I didn't fit in other spaces and have always struggled with my mental health. It has probably informed much of the journey of self-discovery which led me to the world of medicinal and aromatic plants.

So, I signed up to retrain as an aromatherapist, something I'd been thinking about for some time but had always hesitated to do: 'What if this is a waste of time?' and 'What if this turns out to be another dead end?' were questions that kept repeating in my head. But eventually, I had a moment of clarity – my depression had reached a point where I felt I had to do something – the 'sitting on the bedroom floor moment' as I now remember it. The consequences of not doing anything now felt like too much of a risk. So I applied for a career development loan and off I went to the first weekend seminar of my Clinical Aromatherapist Diploma, the first of many that would turn out to be a tonic for my soul and also the beginning of a new way of working. The programme would teach me massage, chemistry, anatomy, physiology and of course, about the healing power of scent. Once I graduated in early 2020, I began my clinical aromatherapy practice and social enterprise, AmberLuna Apothecary, where I now offer herbal workshops, retreats and aroma-based therapies to my community.

It was also at the beginning of 2020 that I applied for a part-time job at the Royal Botanic Gardens, Kew, so that I could begin building an aromatherapy practice on the side. By April, I found myself running the communications team of a programme called Grow Wild that focused on engaging communities and young people across the UK with nature. My relationship with Kew has led me to run staff wellbeing workshops, community outreach programme impact projects, create an online aromatherapy course for the organisation, and to work across various educational and outreach programmes promoting plant science. While working at Kew, I have been fortunate to be able to visit many grassroots community organisations that are doing incredible work to bring people into contact with nature and improve their wellbeing in really creative ways, and I have seen first hand the power that contact with plants can have.

Looking back, my journey to the healing power of scent has in fact been a slow, meandering but definite road. Herbs and aromatherapy have provided a discreet, supportive backdrop throughout my life: I haven't always noticed them, but they've always been there, supporting me through the highs and lows of life. One of my earliest memories is making 'potions' with a childhood friend from the aromatic herbs I had plucked from the garden at my family home. I can still recall the smell of rosemary and thyme as I sat on the ground, mashing them together in a pestle and mortar and mixing in various other flowers. I would leave these concoctions out 'for the fairies' in the garden. I feel that reconnecting with aromatic plants and herbs as an adult has brought me home to who I am, and I'll always be thankful to them for that.

Wherever you are in life, I hope that this book will bring you some of the support, connection, joy and respite that nature, in particular medicinal and aromatic plants, have brought me over the years.

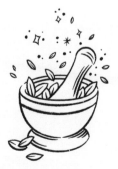

WHAT TO EXPECT FROM THIS BOOK

The Healing Power of Scent is not a guide to the synthetic fragrance ingredients often used in perfumery, which tend to be used for their aromas and don't have any intrinsic therapeutic benefit. Instead this book focuses on aromatics found in the natural world: primarily plants, their essential oils and other natural plant-based ingredients. These are the products that are principally used in aromatherapy, since they have many healing (therapeutic, medicinal) properties.

This book is a journey through the world of aromatic plants (and their non-aromatic friends) – their history, cultural significance and medicinal uses. Along the way, you'll discover the science of our sense of smell and learn some practical ways to harness the power of scent in everyday life. You'll find mindfulness exercises, observation and olfaction (smelling) activities, aromatherapy blends and recipes for skincare products. Throughout, the book aims to explore how we can all learn to better appreciate, respect and harness the benefits that these amazing aromatic materials generously lend us, and how they play a role in supporting our health and wellbeing.

In writing this book, I found myself paying closer attention to the healing aromas around me, and tuning in more frequently to the small details. I felt that the process of creating the activities and researching often brought me a clearer and more mindful connection with the world around me. My hope is that this book will be a resource for you to turn to for mindful, creative and sensory activities, rituals and practices, and that it will help you to develop your own relationships and associations with the aromas and plants within the pages.

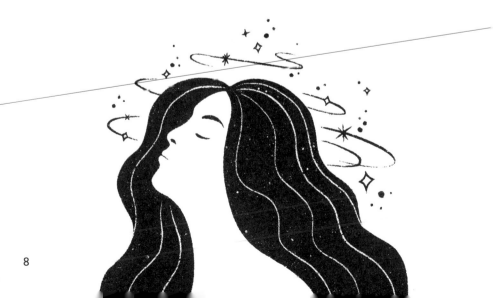

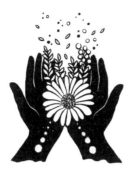

The activities and information have been designed for you to incorporate into your life and hopefully bring an additional dimension to how you experience the world around you. As you meander your way through the pages, recipes and activities, my hope is that it will help you to tap into your inner state, perhaps becoming more attuned to your breathing, emotions and thoughts, and gain some peace, respite, reflection or space from the things that are causing stress or challenging you in life.

Throughout, I've included practical notes to help you make the most of your sensory scent experiences safely and with confidence. I invite you to 'feel' into the activities as much as possible – leaving your 'left brain' (the logical, rational, and planning part) at the door, and to engage with this book with a sense of curiosity, wonder, and openness. Remember: there is no 'right' or 'wrong' in the world of scent – how you experience an aroma may be completely different to how someone else does. That's totally OK – and I'd encourage you to reflect on your own unique experiences and responses to the different aromas as you meet them.

Essential Safety Notes

A guide to using the plant materials and oils described in this book in the safest possible way is given in Chapter 7. Always heed the specific safety advice given in the following recipes and activities, and if in doubt, consult a qualified medical herbalist or aromatherapist.

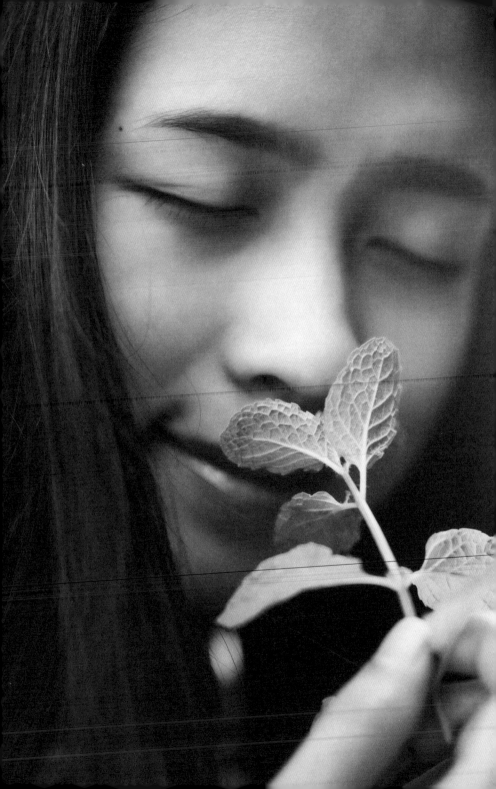

CHAPTER 1

What is Smell?

" Not in the flower
But rather in the nose
The smell resides —
So it seems to me. " Matsuo Bashō, 1694[2]

The poem above, written by 17th-century Japanese poet and Zen Buddhist, Matsuo Bashō, imaginatively and perfectly sums up what we now understand about scent and the sense of smell: the aromatic molecules of a rose may reside within the flower, but it is not until they interact with smell receptors that the aroma can be detected and enjoyed – so the scent only exists in relation to the being that perceives it. This may well be the reason smell is considered the most mysterious and elusive of our senses.

Most of us rely on our sense of smell every day, whether we are aware of it or not, to give us important clues about our surroundings, and to alert us to factors that might have an impact on our wellbeing,[3] such as detecting the smell of burning or a gas leak or inhaling the sweet, calming smell of a pine forest as we wander through it. Did you know that babies can identify their own mothers, just by using their sense of smell?[4] So powerful is this sense, that it has been harnessed by multi-sensory experience designers and marketers worldwide to enhance experiences, stimulate mood changes, and even influence purchasing decisions.[5] Our sense of smell is subtle enough to be able to distinguish between an almost infinite number of chemical compounds, at extremely low concentrations.[6] However, Helen Keller described our sense of smell as the 'fallen angel' of the senses in chapter six of her 1908 collection of essays, *The World I Live In*, and perhaps rightly, suggested that we have 'neglected and disparaged'[7] it. Whilst it may be true that in the West, we typically no longer need to rely on our sense of smell to avoid predation or to forage for berries and mushrooms as our ancestors would have done, and can largely rely on modern technologies for our survival, the more we can understand about how to work with this most mysterious of the senses, the more we can start to embrace it as an integral part of our wellbeing.

The allure and intrigue of our sense of smell, long documented by the likes of Aristotle,[8] Proust[9] and Keller,[10] is undisputed. Perfumers worldwide know the magic that a scent can create. Without a lexicon fit to describe individual aromas, we are forced to use metaphor and descriptive, emotive language such as colour, mood, environment or comparison to flavour in an attempt to pin down a scent's elusive and indescribable character. Natural perfumer, Mandy Aftel, puts it well in her book, *Essence and Alchemy: A Natural History of Perfume*:

> *"Scent reaches us in ways that elude sight and sound but conjure imagination in all its sensuality, unsealing hidden worlds"* [11]

But aroma is not all roses and romanticism. Historically, aroma and smell have been weaponised, primarily by white, western cultures, to actively discriminate against and oppress a wide range of racialised communities and cultural groups, thereby enforcing and maintaining racism and unjust socio-economic hierarchies.[12] It is important to acknowledge this, since it forms an uncomfortable yet undeniable backdrop to our shared cultural history of scent, and examples of it are rife in literature throughout the 19th and 20th centuries, as well as within history itself.

Whilst smell has been harnessed to condemn and oppress, the typical olfactory ability of the average modern westerner is very weak,[13] arguably due to being desensitised to aromas as a society, and living largely in deodorised environments.[14] Research has shown that for certain groups who live in close relationship with the natural world and its smells, aroma can be a much more significant and complex sense than we can understand in Northern Europe. For example, the Desana people of Colombia use the wind to detect 'wind threads'[15] of aroma which tell them information about other nearby tribes when they are travelling, and Umeda people of New Guinea are able to detect even the tiniest traces of fire smoke.[16] They are also known to sleep with aromatic herbs: smell is considered to be directly linked to dreams, and they believe that this practice will bring about 'dreams of a successful hunt'[17] and bring good luck during the hunt itself.[18]

For centuries, herbalists like the 10th-century Persian polymath Avicenna[19] have known the value of aromatics for our health and wellbeing, but only relatively recently have they begun to receive more of the attention they deserve, at least in the West. Respect for, connection to and a deeper understanding of our sense of smell and its complexities has long been overdue a revival, and I hope that this book helps you to reconnect with this forgotten sense to improve your wellbeing, and perhaps brings with it some new and interesting ways for you to experience the world. I also hope that it will provide you with a springboard from which to explore the myriad ways in which scent has influenced, and continues to influence, our lives – be this through our shared cultural history, healing practices around the world, aromatic and sensory practices and environments, and more besides.

"Smell is a potent wizard that transports you across thousands of miles and all the years you have lived. The odors of fruits waft me to my southern home, to my childhood frolics in the peach orchard. Other odors, instantaneous and fleeting, cause my heart to dilate joyously or contract with remembered grief. Even as I think of smells, my nose is full of scents that start awake sweet memories of summers gone and ripening fields far away."

Helen Keller [20]

AROMA DETECTIVES: HOW WE SMELL

We detect smells because they are made up of molecules that are *volatile*. This term, taken from chemistry, describes a substance which has a tendency to evaporate, normally in the form of a vapour.[21] Looking back to its original use, the term was derived from the Latin verb *volare* which means 'to fly', and the noun 'volatile' was widely used in the 14th century to refer to flying creatures such and birds and butterflies.[22] This gives us a clue as to the 'flighty' nature of aromatic substances.

So how do these volatile aromatic substances reach us, and how does our brain know how to interpret each one? Much of our understanding of olfaction, or the process of smelling, remains shrouded in mystery,[23] although in light of the COVID-19 pandemic more research on the respiratory system and olfaction, particularly smell training, is thankfully taking place.[24] The most widely accepted theory of how scent is interpreted by the brain is commonly known as the 'lock and key' theory, first developed in 1949 by R.W. Moncrieff[25] and later developed by John E. Amoore[26] in 1964. Just as each key is unique, and will only fit one lock, the stereo-chemical theory states that olfactory nerve cells are stimulated by different molecules depending on their unique size and shape, or the charge (+/-) of the molecule.[27] This determines which of the various 'slots' on the olfactory receptors the odour molecules will fit into.

Some researchers have suggested an alternative theory, which posits that multiple receptors can recognise several different aromas, much like a combination code system, which would help explain why our olfactory receptors can recognise thousands of unique aromas.[28] We can think of this combination theory as aromatic chords, as in music, as opposed to a single lock and key mechanism. To date, it is still not completely known what causes the lock and key mechanisms to work, despite

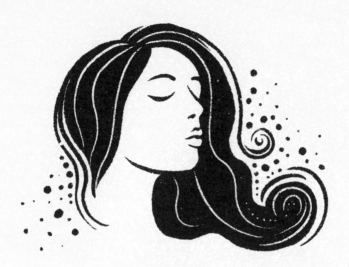

research by a scientist at UCL, Luca Turin, in 1996 which furthered investigations into olfaction even more.[29] Our knowledge is advancing, though, and developments have recently been made by a team of scientists at the University of California, who in March 2023, published a study which, for the first time, shows the 3D structure of a human olfactory receptor protein, and could have exciting implications for the future of our understanding of how receptors and odours bind together to allow us to recognise different aromas.[30]

Aromatic molecules evaporate into the atmosphere and enter the body by way of the nostrils, which are lined with mucus. The molecules dissolve into this substance, and are then detected by specialised receptor cells, which are situated at the end of olfactory neurons, or nerve cells, much like fibres or tiny hairs.[31] These receptors, along with the trigeminal nerve, transmit the signals they receive from different odour molecules to the olfactory bulb, the primary organ of smell, which is made up of nervous tissue.[32] The bulb has a direct link to the brain and will process the nerve impulses before sending them to the olfactory cortex, and then on to parts of the brain that are collectively known as the limbic system.

SCENT AND SENSITIVITY: AROMAS AND THE NERVOUS SYSTEM

Our nervous system is very sensitive to scent. When we detect an aroma, the limbic system, a collection of structures in our brain that includes the thalamus, hypothalamus and amygdala, comes into play. This is the part of our brain which relates to mood and emotion. The amygdala in particular, the first port of call for odours reaching the brain, is concerned with interpreting the 'emotional significance of events in the external world.'[33] Smells have a direct impact on our nervous systems, since inhaling them can trigger the release or inhibition of certain hormones into the bloodstream. These can activate or inhibit our parasympathetic (our 'rest and digest' mode) or sympathetic nervous systems ('fight/flight/freeze') by way of the hypothalamus, which controls our autonomic nervous system, of which the parasympathetic and sympathetic system are the main parts. This influence is due to the scent molecules' direct link to the amygdala and hypothalamus.[34] Current science understands that aroma signals mostly bypass the thalamus,[35] the part of our brain that deals with conscious recognition, and are transmitted straight to the hypothalamus, which has a major influence on the endocrine (hormonal) system. As such, aromas are not always consciously processed by the frontal cortex, where our usual cognition and interpretation occurs,[36] and so the influence aromas have on our body and mind is thought not always to be consciously processed by our brain.

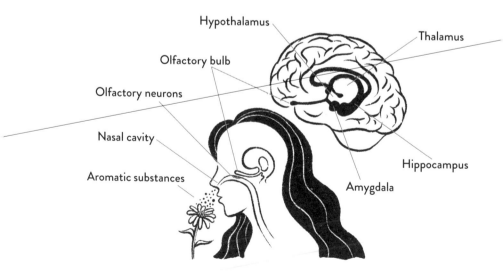

Hypothalamus

Thalamus

Olfactory bulb

Olfactory neurons

Nasal cavity

Hippocampus

Aromatic substances

Amygdala

Anosmia & Smell Training

WHAT IS ANOSMIA?

Anosmia has gained more publicity in recent years due to the COVID-19 outbreak. Upon contracting the virus, many people experience loss of taste (ageusia), smell (anosmia) or both – and some have struggled to recover these senses. Anosmia can occur due to viral infection as with COVID-19, or due to trauma or injury, exposure to harsh chemicals, or certain neurological disorders. Sometimes smell loss is irreversible, but in some cases, smell training can be used to speed up recovery and restore the sense of smell.

WHAT IS SMELL TRAINING?

Smell training has been scientifically shown to help some patients recover their sense of smell. Since essential oils have therapeutic benefits beyond restoring the sense of smell, such as alleviating anxiety, Chrissi Kelly, founder of the now discontinued charity AbScent[37] told me that essential oils are a great tool to use. However, since smells are all around us, we can also make use of our environment to do smell training, providing we don't use harmful chemicals. Scientists and medics alike are now exploring smell training as a way to help patients whose senses have been altered by the COVID-19 virus, with some studies citing excellent results.[38]

HOW TO DO SMELL TRAINING

You'll need a smell-training kit, some patience, and a friend to help you. Smell training requires commitment, although it doesn't take much time out of the day to do. You can purchase one on my AmberLuna website (see Resources and References), which comes with full instructions on how to do smell training as well as a range of essential oil inhalers and herbs or oils to support you in your recovery.

BIOCHEMISTRY AND THE BRAIN:
HOW SCENT INFLUENCES MOOD

The ability of aromas to influence our nervous systems can cause us to feel anger, joy, or fear by altering our biochemistry, impacting both our physical states and mood.[39] To understand how this works on a biochemical level, let's explore the key hormones and brain structures associated with this influence.

AMYGDALA

This structure is part of the limbic system of our brain, and is responsible for mediating emotions such as fear, aggression and anxiety.[40] It does this by sending signals of distress via the nervous system to our adrenal glands, which are located on the top of our kidneys. These glands secrete the hormone epinephrine (adrenaline) and cortisol[41] into our bloodstream[42] which results in stimulation of the sympathetic nervous system, otherwise known as the 'fight or flight' response. When we enter this state, our heart rate increases, sending more blood and oxygen around the body, and our breathing speeds up.[43] This is a natural response to stressful situations and the body's natural way of preparing us to encounter (or run away from) life-threatening situations. However, in conditions like Generalised Anxiety Disorder or chronic stress, this response can activate inappropriately[44] and cause health problems, both physical and psychological.[45] Thankfully, scent can be used to 'teach' the nervous system that it is safe, causing inhibition of the sympathetic nervous system, and activation of the parasympathetic nervous system – our 'rest and digest' mode. Later, we'll explore how this works.

HYPOTHALAMUS

This brain structure is also part of the limbic system and is responsible for the release or inhibition of hormones. Hormones (including dopamine, the 'feel-good' or 'pleasure' hormone)[46] [47] are released into the bloodstream and go on to stimulate the pituitary gland to produce more hormones (such as oxytocin, the 'love hormone')[48] which influence our thyroid and adrenal glands, reproductive system and autonomic nervous system.[49] Since the hypothalamus is the area 'where the nervous system and endocrine [hormonal] system overlap',[50] this cascade of hormones can have an impact on anything from our mood, to our sleep and metabolism.[51]

CLINICAL AROMATHERAPY RESEARCH IN PRACTICE

Several research studies and systematic reviews have demonstrated the positive effects of different aromas on mood disorders like depression,[52] noted improvements in cognitive function in mice, suggesting that aromatherapy could be an effective treatment for Alzheimer's disease,[53] and recorded reduced stress levels in teenagers within academic environments.[54] Anxiety in dental waiting rooms has been abated by aromatherapy,[55] menopausal anxiety and depression have been relieved,[56] and it has been shown to 'significantly decrease'[57] labour pain and anxiety. Midwives in the UK do, on occasion and with appropriate training and experience, offer aromatherapy through inhalation and massage to their pregnant patients – this is perhaps the most widely accepted form of aromatherapy within mainstream healthcare contexts like the NHS (National Health Service, UK), probably due to its efficacy[58] and relative safety.[59]

Aromatherapy has also been shown to improve postpartum 'depression, fatigue, sleep quality, pain after caesarean-delivery and post-episiotomy pain'[60] and reduce dysmenorrhea, too, so it is a useful and gentle tool for those who are pregnant or postpartum people to carry all the way through their pregnancy, birth and on into parenthood. In my aromatherapy clinic, for example, I offer a specialised workshop for parents-to-be, which includes a bespoke pregnancy massage tutorial, and a series of customised inhalation and massage oil blends for the three trimesters, as well as specific blends for use during labour. I also provide follow-up information and postpartum products, such as balms or oil blends, if the clients prefer. My clients and I have found this to be an enjoyable, holistic and gentle approach to ensuring that parents and their birth partners feel supported throughout their pregnancy. Treatment can normally be given alongside and in respect of ongoing treatment or appointments within mainstream healthcare.

Memories of Scent

*"Our senses connect us intimately to the past, connect us in
ways that most of our cherished ideas never could"*

Diane Ackerman, *A Natural History of the Senses*[61]

As well as their neurological and hormonal effects, aromas can influence our mood through memories and associations. Have you ever been walking down the street, and caught a scent on the breeze that immediately transported you back in time, or to a cherished place from your childhood? For me, the smell of eucalyptus has always transported me back to a park on the coast in Tasmania, Australia, where I lived for a year when I was eight years old. Not only is the scent strongly associated with a sense of place, but the colours, textures and sounds, even the breeze and temperature, come clearly into my mind's eye. When I inhale the resinous, baked and distinctive aroma of the leaves as the sun gently warms them and releases their oils, I picture the park swings, the chipped bark underfoot, and the afternoon light on the wet rocks and dancing across the ocean. I can almost see the seabirds fishing, and feel the breeze and sunlight on my skin.

So why is scent such a powerful and seemingly magical conjurer when it comes to memory? It's all to do with the limbic system again. In her 1938 novel, *Rebecca*, Daphne du Maurier's protagonist wishes:

*" If only there could be an invention that
bottled up a memory, like scent. And
it never faded, and it never got stale.
And then, when one wanted it, the bottle
could be uncorked, and it would be like
living the moment all over again. "*

Daphne du Maurier, *Rebecca*[62]

In fact, we already have access to this invention: scent is the key to the revival of vivid memories. The brain's limbic system, in addition to regulating mood and emotion, is also responsible for the creation of memory associations. More specifically, the hippocampus, which is the area of the brain that converts short-term memory to long-term memory.[63] In a 2020 talk, 'Olfaction in Science and Society', sponsored by the Harvard Museum of Natural History, Dawn Goldworm, co-founder of an olfactive branding company, 12.29, explains:

" . . . smell and emotion are stored as one memory and childhood is usually the time of life in which you create the basis for smells you will like and hate for the rest of your life."[64]

While not bottled, these scent-memories are contained subconsciously within the brain's anterior olfactory nucleus,[65] and are 'uncorked' when triggered by a certain evocative scent. The smell of mown grass, lavender laundry water in a grandmother's garden, campfire woodsmoke on a cherished holiday, pine disinfectant on freshly-scrubbed bathroom floors, cedar moth repellent in an old wardrobe, seaweed drying in the sun, and toasting bread in a family home are all scent-memories that students on my aromatherapy and herbalism workshops and retreats have recalled when I have asked which aromas evoke memory responses for them. For some people, the same aroma will have a range of responses, and they can differ wildly! Just as no two lives are alike, it is seldom that two people will have the same associations with a particular scent.

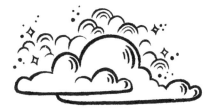

MAKING NEW MEMORIES

While most scent-memory associations may be crafted and cemented during childhood, as adults we do have the ability to influence, change and create new associations.[66] As a practising aromatherapist, before beginning a treatment, I make sure to ask my clients whether there are any aromas they know they absolutely cannot bear so that I avoid triggering any negative scent-memory-emotion responses, and I try to use essential oils and extracts with which they have already formed positive associations. For example, if a client is working with a particular challenge, such as insomnia, we might work together through the course of our treatments to create new aroma-memory associations. Since our brains are plastic[67] (they can learn, adapt and change), and have the amazing ability to form new scent associations through 'induce[d] emotional olfactory learning',[68] aromatherapists are uniquely placed to support their clients to create and build an association between the scent of German chamomile (*Matricaria recutita*) and lavender (*Lavandula angustifolia*), for example. The relaxing, dimly-lit ambience and safe, therapeutic space that the treatment room provides will further enhance this association. Since odours 'vividly trigger the evocation of emotional experiences',[69] over the course of regular consultations and treatments, we can build a trusting, therapeutic relationship and work together to strengthen and reinforce the message we are sending to the client's brain. The aromas of German chamomile and lavender in combination with a soothing massage treatment, a warm, calming space and a listening ear, is effectively telling their brain 'I'm safe', 'I can relax', 'I can feel calm and happy' and 'it's time to sleep'.

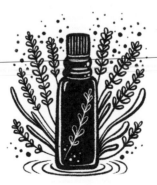

What's more, the client is then able to take a blend of these aromatic oils with them when they leave the treatment space, by way of an inhaler, roll-on oil blend, or room spray, which with time and practice, will enable them to conjure up the new, positive association when they are struggling to sleep or experiencing high levels of stress, and will have a positive, relaxing effect on their nervous system, emotions and muscles.[70] This is what is known as a 'learned odour response'[71] and can easily and effectively be employed in a number of different scenarios to elicit 'measurable effects on cognitive performance, stress, and mood'.[72]

Olfactory Fatigue

In her book, *Fragrant: The Secret Life of Scent,* Mandy Aftel mentions a phenomenon known as 'olfactory fatigue' whereby the overstimulation of our olfactory organ can distort and weaken our ability to perceive different aromas.[73] Have you ever tried smelling samples of perfume, or flowers, only to find that after a while you can no longer detect the different notes and aromas? Or perhaps all the scents start to smell the same? This is olfactory fatigue. Contrary to popular belief, smelling coffee beans will not 'reset your nose', and actually, Aftel argues, smelling something made out of wool might be a better alternative. Science and food author Harold McGee, in his book *Nose Dive,* states that lanolin, the waxy coating found on wool, 'holds' onto aromas.[74] Perhaps this is why wool works well as a sort of 'olfactory reset button'.

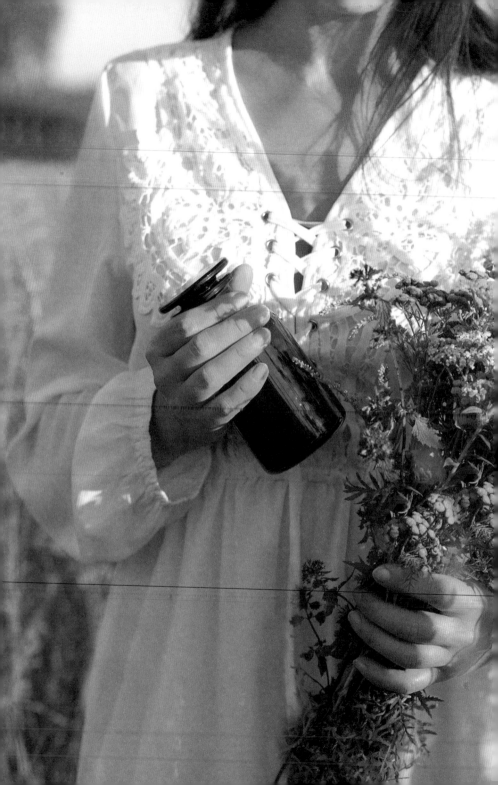

CHAPTER 2

What is Aromatherapy?

"Aromatherapy is shamanism for everyone" Kurt Schnaubelt[75]

Aromatherapy is a branch of herbalism, which means the practice of using medicinal plants in various ways to both treat and prevent disease. From the Unani Tibb system of Avicenna's time,[76] to Ayurveda in ancient India,[77] Traditional Chinese Medicine[78] to Traditional Western Herbal Medicine,[79] many cultures have developed their own herbal medicine practices which are now several thousands of years old, and still inform and contribute significantly to our modern medical practices: digoxin, ephedrine and aspirin are all examples of this.[80] It is important to acknowledge that Traditional Western Herbalism derives its roots from many cultures and sources, including ancient Greek medicine of Hippocrates' time, as well as Native American herbalism[81] and African (Egyptian) traditions.[82]

Aromatic plants have been recorded as being used for perfumery and mummification as early as around 3100BCE in ancient Egypt,[83] where frankincense and myrrh were key aromatics[84] and herbs such as meadowsweet (*Filipendula ulmaria*) were used to strew the floors in homes in the West in the Middle Ages.[85] As we will explore in Chapter 3, aromatherapy emerged as a discipline from the discovery and development of distillation between the 8th to 10th centuries in the Middle East[86] whereby aromatic steam was captured and perfumes or ointments produced[87] ultimately leading to the production of our well-loved essential oils.

Unique in their rich, intoxicating aromas, their elusiveness and instability, natural essences became highly prized and made their way all over the world via the silk, spice and other trade routes, by sea and caravan.[88] It is important to note that much of this trade happened during the Age of Exploration (perhaps better termed as the Age of Exploitation) where European traders, notably Dutch and English companies, colonised and exploited the countries that were the principal producers and exporters of many of these aromatic products.[89] Slavery, along with the cotton, tea and sugar trades would later take the place of the spice trade.[90]

Today, raw aromatic substances from plants are still used in perfumery, as well as in religious, spiritual and ceremonial settings. Frankincense resin is burned in churches for blessing a space,[91] and palo santo, a sacred, and now endangered South American wood, is used by shamans to dispel negative energy and more besides. In Japan, *Koh-do*, which translates as 'the way of incense', is a ceremonial practice and art that focuses on listening to what a given aroma may have to tell the participant, and allows them to both appreciate and play with a variety of scents.[92]

But these more spiritual and aesthetic practices of using plant aromatics differ quite substantially from how they are used therapeutically in aromatherapy clinic rooms. The modern practice of aromatherapy in the West involves harnessing the therapeutic properties of the aromatic plants, which are held in their essential oils, and requires the prior distillation of the plants. Blends of these oils are applied in an intelligent, targeted way to produce a particular therapeutic effect, whether emotional or physical, by a trained therapist. By reading this book, you will come to understand more about the therapeutic uses, qualities and energies of some of the key essential oils in the aromatherapist's toolkit, which will equip you to safely and successfully experience the healing power of scent for yourself.

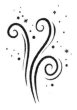

Disclaimer: This book is not a professional training manual and therefore does not equip you to treat other people in a professional context. Professional aromatherapists undergo rigorous training before they are able to treat clients. You should take care when preparing treatments for yourself, adhere to safety guidelines and consult a professional aromatherapist and/or medical herbalist if you are unsure about anything.

Energetic Medicine

Many systems of traditional herbal medicine use an energetics-based approach to treatment. These theories link diseases, herbs and people with one or more of the elements, humours or qualities shown in the diagram below. This diagram shows the Traditional Western approach: Galen's humoral system of medicine, combined with Aristotle's four elements theory. Each season, element, and period of life corresponds to a particular quality, and similarly each herb or essential oil has energetic qualities that make it more or less appropriate for the treatment of a specific illness or imbalance. So, a herb or oil is either cooling, drying, heating or moistening,[93] and should be chosen carefully to counteract the imbalance of the disease. In practical terms, you may choose to use lavender essential oil as part of an inhalation blend for someone who is experiencing insomnia and hot flushes at night, since it is considered a cooling, drying herb and hot flushes are a hot, damp condition, energetically speaking. Chinese medicine uses the five elements of fire, earth, metal, water and wood, whereas Ayurveda focuses on the three doshas: Kapha, Pitta and Vata. There are some overlaps between the general principles of the various theories, and lots of great books on humoral and energetic medicine are available (see Resources and References).

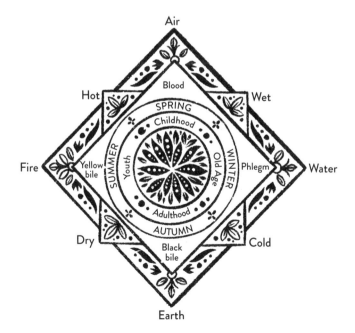

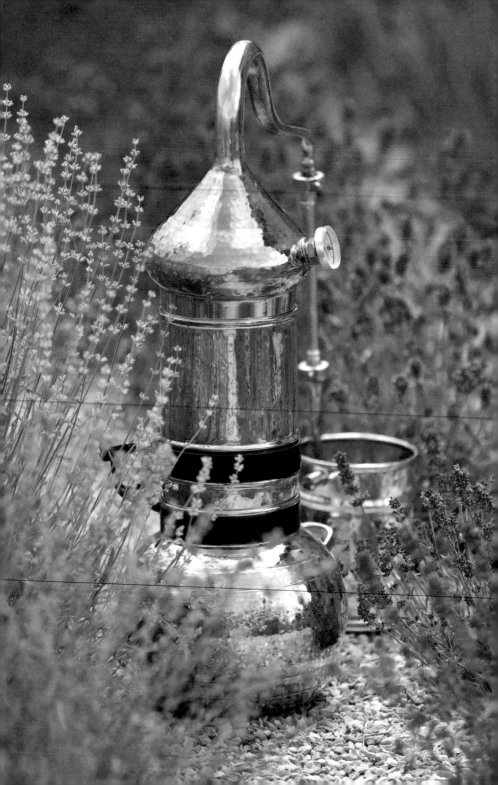

CHAPTER 3

Scent for Therapeutic Effect

"... The odour arising from what is fragrant, that odour which is pleasant in its own right, is, so to say, always beneficial to persons in any state of bodily health whatever." Aristotle[94]

We have explored how scent molecules enter our brain and bloodstream, and discovered that they can influence our biology, from our mood to our physical state. But what does this mean in practice, when working with scent in a therapeutic way? In other words, how do we channel these aromatic molecules and work with them, in order to produce the most beneficial wellbeing and health effects, and generate our intended outcome? It starts with understanding a little more about organic chemistry and how aromatic therapeutic substances are extracted and produced, as well as being clear about what effect we are intending to have on the body, whether it may be physical or emotional.

Aromatics in Aromatherapy

As I write, the smell of sweet orange, *Citrus × sinensis* drifts across the room and almost immediately fills my head with a summery, sharp, and uplifting feeling that I know only this particular aroma provokes in me. This glorious fruit is a hybrid between a mandarin and a pomelo, and creates a unique aroma profile as a result.[95] Earlier, I peeled the rind from a big bag of oranges, and am now dehydrating it, to preserve for future herbal tea-blending endeavours. Within the peel of an orange, tiny aromatic molecules are stored. Have you ever looked closely at the skin of an orange? Chances are you have noticed small, circular 'dots' that cover the peel. These dots are actually cells, or glands[96] that contain the aromatic oil, or essential oil, that bursts with the familiar orangey scent. Squeeze a section of orange rind between two fingers, with a piece of tissue held behind it, and you will likely notice the oil as it sprays out of the broken cells and onto the paper. You might even notice that the oil has a colour, often a pale yellow-orange.

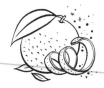

The Anatomy of an Aromatic Molecule

If we were to look at the oil droplets from orange peel on a molecular level, we'd notice that most of the aromatic molecules in orange peel are small, even more so than others. Around 85% of the molecules responsible for the citrussy smell[97] (citronellal, geranial, neral and limonene) are tiny. They are monoterpenoids, meaning they have just ten atoms of carbon per molecule.[98 99] Chemically speaking, this is minuscule in both size and weight and explains how the scent instantly travels across the room, up my nostrils and makes me feel as if I'm on a sunshine holiday in the Mediterranean. The smaller and lighter the molecule, the more volatile it is, and the faster it can reach our olfactory system, brain and bloodstream.[100] This makes plants containing monoterpenes extremely useful, both for inhalation blends and in topical products since their volatility[101] and small size,[102] lend themselves well to both treatment methods.

WHAT IS AN ESSENTIAL OIL?

Essential oils belong to a group of plant chemicals known as secondary metabolites.[103] While not essential for a plant's survival *per se*,[104] secondary metabolites are multifunctional phytochemicals (plant chemicals) that as well as protecting the plant from infection or predation, attracting pollinators or aiding in seed dispersal,[105] have medicinal properties that we can benefit from as humans. In the case of essential oils, this includes antibacterial, antiviral and antifungal actions, amongst others.[106] These oils are an extremely concentrated mix of plant chemicals, many of which are also aromatic. This is where we get the term 'aromatherapy' from – although as you'll come to learn, it's not just the nice smell that has a therapeutic effect!

An essential oil may be produced in various parts of the plant, depending on the reason for its presence. This could include the peel of the fruit, as in our previous sweet orange example, or within the flowers, stems, leaves, bark, root and buds of a wide range of shrubs, herbs and flowering plants. They can even be found within the resins and heartwood of some tree species.[107]

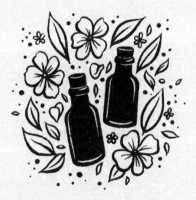

CATEGORISING ESSENTIAL OILS

In her book, *The Fragrant Mind*, Valerie Ann Worwood categorises essential oils into nine personality groups: Florals, Fruities, Herbies, Leafies, Resinies, Rooties, Seedies, Spicies and Woodies. Whilst subjective, these groups are helpful as a starting point for getting to know our *Materia Aromatica*. Not only do they tell us more about the parts of the plant that a given essential oil predominantly comes from, but they are also an interesting way of working with the oils therapeutically. By associating each essential oil group with a dominating personality type, according to Worwood, treatment of emotional imbalances can become more effective. She believes that if we can find out which group (or groups) of oils a client tends to be particularly drawn to, we can harness the 'relationship between particular people and particular oils'[108] to improve physical, emotional and spiritual outcomes. Below is a chart that details some examples of popular essential-oil producing plants, and explains which part of the plant the oils are extracted from. I'm always amazed by the variety of ways plants find to protect themselves or ensure their longevity as a species – and that in doing so, they're able to produce such a wonderful variety of complex fragrances, too.

PART OF PLANT	EXAMPLE OIL	LATIN NAME
Flower	Rose	*Rosa x damascena*
Pericarp (rind)	Bergamot	*Citrus x bergamia*
Fruits (berries)	Black pepper	*Piper nigrum*
Leaves	Geranium	*Pelargonium graveolens*
Aerial parts of plant	Melissa	*Melissa officinalis*
Resin (gum or sap)	Myrrh	*Commiphora myrrha*
Rhizome	Ginger (rhizome)	*Zingiber officinale*
Seed	Coriander	*Coriandrum sativum*
Bark	Cinnamon	*Cinnamomum verum*
Wood	Cedar	*Cedrus atlantica*

Sources: Data from 'Plants of the World Online', Royal Botanic Gardens, Kew 2022; and Robert Tisserand and Rodney Young, *Essential Oil Safety*, 2nd ed (see Resources and References).

The Essence of a Plant?

As we have already touched on with the example of *Citrus x sinensis* (sweet orange), essential oils are made up of very small, volatile molecules, often of between just 10-15 carbon atoms in size.[109] They are oils, but not in the sense with which we might be familiar, such as the non-volatile 'fixed' or 'carrier' oils used in cooking, like coconut or olive oil, for example. The clue is in their name. The naming of these extracts as 'essential oils' is thought to be derived from *quinta essentia*, a Latin term given by 16th-century physician Paracelsus, designating the oils as the 'quintessence' or 'fifth element'[110] of plants that he studied.[111] 'Essential' in the modern context refers not to the idea that the oil is essential for the plant's survival or growth, nor that it is necessarily the true essence of the plant (although this is debatable from a more energetic or spiritual standpoint – indeed, some renowned aromatherapists state that the scent makes a 'vital contribution to [the plant's] natural healing properties').[112] Scientifically speaking, the term 'essential oil' means that the oil evaporates – or is volatile – at room temperature.[113]

Essential oils share some of the physical properties of our more familiar cooking or non-volatile oils: they do not mix well with water. In other words, they tend to be insoluble in water (hydrophobic). Their lipophilic (fat-soluble) nature means that they have a propensity for dissolving in fats and other oils. They are also soluble in solvents such as ethanol (alcohol).[114] This means that aromatherapists and natural product formulators need to choose their preparation methods carefully when it comes to creating products and blends.

Distillation: The Art of Extraction

Essential oils are secreted by glandular trichomes (tiny hairs) on[115] or oil sacs within[116] the plant. In order to extract them, it is necessary to break or rupture the oil glands or sacs. This can be done in a number of ways. In aromatherapy, there are two methods that are largely accepted as suitable for therapeutic purposes, since they don't require harsh chemicals to extract the essential oils. They are based on the ancient technique of distillation, or a more simple method known as cold expression. The way a plant is extracted largely depends on the 'yield' or amount of essential oil it contains, and how susceptible the plant is to being damaged by heat or oxidation.[117]

The discovery of steam distillation is largely attributed to 10th century Persian polymath, Ibn Sīnā,[118] or Avicenna as he is known in the West. His pioneering technique for the extraction of essential oils, in particular attar of rose, probably *Rosa × damascena*, or Mohammadi rose,[119] arguably revolutionised herbal medicine and aromatherapy. He invented the copper coil that cools the distillate and allows for the condensation of the essential oil and the aromatic water. This technique, still employed today, was subsequently used to produce both alcoholic drinks and essential oils, and was a pioneering scientific discovery at the time, since until that point aromatic substances, including herbal medicines, were simply made from mixtures of oil and crushed herbs or petals.[120]

In the UK, essential oil distillation is a mid- to large-scale industrial process and is usually carried out on-site at farms or at specialised production units, although smaller stills do exist. Even tiny stove-top apparatuses are available to purchase for the distillation of aromatic waters and essential oils at home.

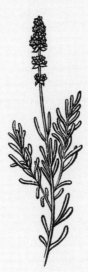

Across Europe, at sites where aromatic medicinal plants have historically been grown, harvested and processed, working or display copper stills can still be found. In the 1600s, the town of Grasse, France, was a hotbed of the leather and tanning industry, but in a bid to cover up the stench of lye and animals, leather glove makers began to scent their products with the extracts of aromatic plants, which grow plentifully in the Mediterranean climate. As a result, the area eventually became much more famous for its fragrance industry than its leather![121] Even today, it remains a popular destination for scent tourism and there are perfumeries and museums dedicated to fragrance. Distillery tours, perfumery workshops and scented garden visits all abound to whet the appetite of the aromatically-curious traveller.

Norfolk, England, is home to some of the most famous lavender fields in the UK, and during my aromatherapy diploma training I was lucky enough to visit a small, family-run working essential oil production farm, Norfolk Essential Oils, as well as the Norfolk Lavender fields and gardens, on a class day-trip. At both locations, during the peak of high summer, my coursemates, tutors and I observed both steam and hydrodistillation techniques. At the farm, we observed modern industrial harvesting techniques and stills, and at the gardens, we saw a traditional copper still demonstration in full swing, a member of the garden staff explaining the process from start to finish, adding big forkfuls of freshly-harvested lavender to a tall stack ready for processing, as we inhaled the rich, sweet aroma.

Modern Methods of Extraction

While the recollection of my Norfolk experience paints a rather idyllic, sensory and romantic view of distillation, Aromatherapists today typically rely on larger-scale industrial methods for the production of our precious oils. Below, I've detailed the most commonly-used processes used today. Bear in mind that not all extraction methods are suitable for therapeutic purposes since they require some harsh chemicals, traces of which are sometimes left behind in the oils and hydrosols (aromatic waters).

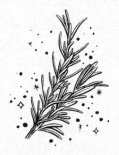

STEAM AND HYDRODISTILLATION

These are the two extraction methods most commonly associated with the production of essential oils for therapeutic use. In hydrodistillation, plant material is submerged in water, in a container which is connected to a tube above. Heat is then applied from beneath the vessel, and the oil sacs or trichomes are ruptured by the heat. The water and essential oil molecules contained within the plant are subsequently converted into steam and evaporate, passing up, and into the tube. With steam distillation, the process is very similar, except that the plant material is suspended above the water, rather than submerged in it, and the steam passes up through the plant matter.

The now-vapourised oil and steam are passed along the tube into a condensing chamber, which is composed of a second large vessel, filled with cold water. As with the traditional stills of Avicenna's time, the oil and steam pass slowly through a coiled metal (traditionally copper) tube within the cold water condenser, allowing the mixture to condense back into essential oil and water.

Essential oils and water have different densities and polarities: Oils are lipophilic (more likely to be fat-soluble), whereas water, and some water-soluble molecules that are extracted in the distillation process, are hydrophilic (more likely to be water-soluble), so when the oil and aromatic water pass into their final chamber, a separator, the substances separate naturally. The essential oil floats on top of the aromatic water (hydrosol, or hydrolat), where it is then tapped off and bottled ready for distribution.

Steam distillation is considered a more intensive method of extraction than hydrodistillation, and as such is mainly used for plants which are able to tolerate more heat without their oil quality being compromised. This typically includes woodier herbs like rosemary (*Salvia rosmarinus*). Hydrodistillation is gentler and is more often used to produce essential oils from herbs that contain more thermolabile (destroyed or damaged in heat) molecules, such as basil (*Ocimum basilicum*) leaves, or the rhizome of ginger (*Zingiber officinale*).[122] It also has the added benefit that it allows plant matter like rose petals or powdered herbs to be separated and extracted more easily – they have a tendency to stick together in steam distillation.[123]

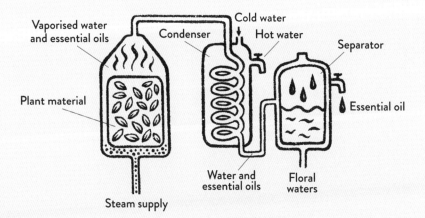

Vaporised water
and essential oils

Condenser

Cold water

Hot water

Separator

Plant material

Essential oil

Water and
essential oils

Floral
waters

Steam supply

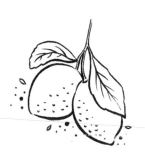

COLD EXPRESSION

This method of extracting essential oils is only used for extracting the essential oils from citrus fruits, and since heat is not involved, it allows the oil to retain a strong aroma which is akin to that of the fresh fruit.[124] These fruits hold their essential oils in the pericarp (skin) of the fruit, near the surface, in glands or sacs. As such, distillation is not required to extract the oil. The fruit, including the peel, is passed through a mechanical apparatus which crushes the peel and releases the volatile oil, which is then released as an emulsion along with water, juice and other molecules from the fruit. This emulsion is then passed through a high-speed centrifuge which separates the essential oil from the aromatic water and juice, and allows it to be tapped off.[125]

SOLVENT EXTRACTION

Alternative methods for the production of aromatic plant extracts include solvent-based extraction processes. Although technically they don't produce true essential oils, the resulting products are still used therapeutically, and in cosmetics or skincare. Two of the most commonly used solvent extraction methods include supercritical CO_2 extraction, which produces CO_2 extracts, and hexane extraction, which produces a product known as an 'absolute'.[126] The advantage of CO_2 extraction is that it requires much less heat than distillation, and therefore does not damage the heat-sensitive (thermolabile) aromatic molecules.[127] However, it does require specialised equipment, since the carbon dioxide must be highly pressurised in order to extract aromatic oils. As a result, CO_2 extracts tend to be more expensive than essential oils.

Hexane extraction is also very effective at distilling a wider range of aromatics than steam or hydrodistillation, and the product (the absolute) typically contains a wider range of organic chemicals. Typically, an absolute will have a much stronger aroma than an essential oil from the same plant. However, since it requires the use of hexane (a compound often added to petroleum), many aromatherapists prefer not to use absolutes for therapeutic purposes[128] as traces of the solvent often remain in them.

Sweet Floral Waters

Hydrolats, hydrosols or aromatic waters are names given to the water which is produced at the end of the essential oil extraction process in hydro- or steam distillation. While technically a by-product of the process, since the main aim is to extract the essential oils, these waters are medicinal and therapeutic in their own right. They contain some of the more water-soluble plant molecules that are not present in the essential oils. Fragrant, light and fresh, hydrosols of neroli, or orange blossom (*Citrus aurantium* var. *amara* flos.), lavender (*Lavandula angustifolia*) and rose (*Rosa × damascena*) are all commonly-used hydrosols in my treatment room, and have their place alongside their oil counterparts in therapeutic treatments. Depending on the herb used, these gentle aromatics can be applied topically as mild, astringent skin toners, used as a mist to cool and refresh the body, drunk in aromatic herbal teas or cool drinks alongside fresh, edible botanicals, or even combined into therapeutic skin creams.

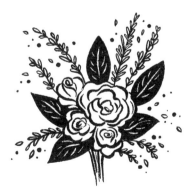

Capturing the Elusive: Traditional Aroma Extraction Methods

Scent is notoriously elusive. Writers, scientists and more recently cultural heritage researchers[129] have attempted to describe, capture and preserve some of our most evocative, interesting and culturally-important aromas, with varying degrees of success. Only relatively recently are we beginning to learn how we might preserve some of these mysterious and flighty molecules for the long term. While modern methods for capturing scent are continuously evolving, some of our oldest and most basic techniques are still used, and are among the most accessible for the home aroma explorer.

" Scents were like rain, or birds. They left and came back. They told you their own stories, letting you know when the tide was low or the oatmeal was done cooking or the apple trees were getting ready to bloom. But they never stayed."

Erica Bauermeister, *The Scent Keeper*[130]

ENFLEURAGE

A traditional method of scent extraction with its roots in Ancient Egypt,[131] enfleurage is a labour-intensive and expensive process which is only used occasionally nowadays.[132] The technique works particularly well with expensive florals such as jasmines (*Jasminum sambac* and *Jasminum grandiflorum*) rose (*Rosa × damascena*) or tuberose (*Agave amica*). Non-aromatic semi solid animal fats[133] like tallow or lard would be spread on glass plates, and flower petals spread across the fat (the chassis[134]) and laid to rest and infuse for around 24 hours.[135] This process would be repeated, with the same fat, up to 36 times[136] to infuse it with the rich, sensual aromas of the delicate flowers. Once saturated with the flowers' perfume, the aromatic pomade (aromatic fat) would be washed with alcohol to extract the aroma. Due to the process being completely 'natural' and free from heat, it is still considered one of the purest forms of aromatic extraction, hence the high price point.

MACERATION

Another ancient and less labour-intensive technique than enfleurage is maceration. This technique is still used by aromatherapists and herbalists[137] to extract medicinal and aromatic properties from plants today, since it is so accessible and effective. Essentially, this means adding an aromatic herb like lavender (*Lavandula angustifolia*) to a base (carrier) oil[138] such as sweet almond (*Prunus amygdalus* var. *dulcis*) until it softens, and the medicinal and aromatic compounds are extracted. For small quantities, fresh or dried herbs are usually chopped and added to an airtight, sterilised jar, and left on a sunny windowsill for up to a month. The gentle heat of the sunlight will rupture the essential oil glands and release them along with other medicinal plant constituents into the carrier, leaving you with a beautifully-scented oil that can be used topically for massage, for example. It is worth noting that if fresh herbs are used, they will contain water, and combining oil with water can lead to microbial growth, so it is advisable to dry the herbs first if you plan to try this yourself – unless you know how to formulate using natural preservatives in the correct way.

DRYING HERBS

I use a dehydrator on a low setting to dry my herbs at home, adjusting the temperature depending on how much water they contain, but there are lots of other ways to do it if you don't have access to a dehydrator. A fan oven set to between 30-50°C (85-120°F) works just as well if you're pushed for time. Check the temperature regularly to make sure the plants don't go brown or 'cook' – an hour or two should be plenty for most flowers or leafy herbs. Another, longer way I was taught by a friend is to put aromatic herbs in an old pair of clean tights, and hang them in a well-ventilated, cool, dry place until they are crisp and completely dry. Inevitably, by heating or leaving the plants to dry, some of the 'fresher' volatile oils will evaporate and the aromas slightly changed or lost, but they will still make lovely therapeutic products that you can enjoy.

Safety Notes

Take care when selecting your herbs, never consume your macerated oils and consult the safety advice in Chapter 7. Some recommended further reading on herbs and aromatherapy can be found at the end of this book (see Resources and References).

Sourcing Essential Oils

Many of my workshop participants and clients ask me about where to source essential oils and aromatic products. There is no straightforward answer to this question, since the world of aromatherapy and essential oil regulation and production is complex and falls under multiple pieces of legislation (in the UK).

The Aromatherapy Trade Council is an independent body which offers guidance to professionals on sourcing essential oils, and also provides up-to-date information on legislation. You can find the link to their website in the Resources and References section at the back of this book.

As a general rule, I try to apply the following principles to ensure that as far as possible, I procure oils from well-managed, small production farms or suppliers who work closely with small-scale farmers. I prefer to use organically and sustainably produced oils wherever possible.

› Speak with your supplier. This will help you understand more about their employment and farming or production processes. A good supplier will be able to provide information on their supply chain, organic status and extraction methods. If you want to get more scientific about it, you can often request the GCMS (Gas Chromatography Mass Spectrometry analysis)[139] results for a particular oil from your supplier which show a breakdown of the chemistry of the oil.

› Buy sustainably. For me, this means buying organic and small-scale wherever possible. As with food, organic status means that there will be strict rules about how producers can grow and process their products. Since the oils I use therapeutically will be applied to the skin and inhaled, I prefer to use organic oils if I can. In terms of preserving soil, plant and human health, organic is also preferable. Whilst I am not here to try to convince anyone about the benefits of organic growing, you can find a link to the Soil Association website in the Resources and References section if you'd like to learn more. Supporting smaller producers can mean a greater degree of visibility regarding the production from plant to bottle, but again it's wise to speak with the supplier to understand how they work and if you wish to support them. I wrote an article for *Herbal Reality* on essential oils and sustainability,[140] which you can also find in the resources section if you'd like to read more on sustainability.

› Buy only what you need. Essential oils, like with any natural product, have a shelf life. Typically this can range from one to three years if the oils are stored correctly (in a cool, dark place and in airtight glass bottles). Buying in bulk, unless you're planning to make industrial amounts of bath oil or face cream, won't really save you any money, since the contents might oxidise before you have the chance to use it all. It can be tempting to invest in hundreds of bottles of different oils, but if you buy a little, and replace as needed, you'll spread the cost and reduce waste too. Buying one or two oils at a time is also a good way to build a relationship with each plant, each oil, as you develop your knowledge and understanding of their characters and properties.

Aromatherapy for Wellbeing: The Power of Plants for Emotional and Physical Health

In the sections titled 'Scent and Sensitivity: aromas and the nervous system' and 'Biochemistry and the Brain: how scent influences mood', we explored how essential oils have an impact on our mood by stimulating the release of certain hormones that influence our autonomic nervous system, and we looked at how our sense of smell is directly connected to our brain via the olfactory bulb.

INHALATION FOR EMOTIONAL WELLBEING

It is thanks to this direct link to the brain and an aroma's ability to influence our nervous system that aromatherapy is so helpful for emotional regulation and wellbeing. Inhaling essential oils is the quickest and most direct route to influencing our nervous system,[141] so it stands to reason that this is the most commonly used method by aromatherapists if they are trying to produce a certain emotional effect when treating a client. There are a number of ways to prepare blends of essential oils for inhalation which can be chosen based on the context, specific need, or availability. Later on, you'll find some ideas for blends for emotional wellbeing that can be used with some of these methods.

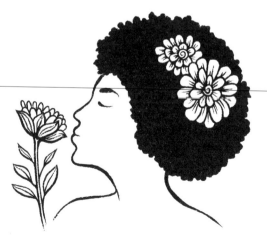

TISSUES

Perhaps the simplest way to inhale essential oils, but one of the most effective for short-term use is on a facial tissue. In my treatment room, I usually apply four or five drops of a blend of essential oils to a tissue which the client can tuck into the massage couch cover and inhale during their treatment, enjoying the psychological effects that the blend produces, along with the physiological benefits provided by the massage and topical oil blend. This is a really easy way to use aromatherapy discreetly when out and about, since you can keep it in a pocket and have it to hand to inhale when needed. Similarly, the tissue can be put inside a pillowcase to aid sleep (although the oils should not come into direct contact with the skin).

NEBULISERS AND VAPOURISERS

These are electronic devices which emit gentle puffs of essential oil into the room. Usually left on for between 30 minutes to an hour, they are a subtle yet powerful way to use aromatherapy within a room. I often fragrance my treatment room or study with a calming blend of oils prior to starting work. Nebulisers usually have a reservoir where a small amount of undiluted essential oil is added, and is atomised into smaller droplets and forced out of the nebuliser by air at a high pressure, dispersing the aroma into the space. A vapouriser usually has a reservoir where water is added, along with a few drops of essential oil, which is then vibrated using ultrasonic waves. This creates microscopic particles of oils which then spread into the air.

TEA LIGHT DIFFUSERS

Tea light diffusers work by using heat to gently warm a water reservoir from underneath, to which a few drops of essential oil is added. As the heat warms the water and oil, the steam and aromatic molecules evaporate into the room, and distribute their fragrance. This is also a lovely way to add ambience to a room, although it is considered less effective therapeutically than nebulisers or vapourisers.

ROLL-ONS

While it is also a topical form of application, an oil roll-on can be used as an inhalation blend, too. It is a convenient and pocket-sized way to carry a blend of several oils with you throughout the day. Usually diluted to a safe percentage in a base (carrier) oil, the essential oils can be applied to the wrists or temples, and massaged to warm them and release their aromas. Then they can be inhaled at the same time as being absorbed into the bloodstream through the skin.

STEAM INHALATIONS

Although this method is most often used for treating respiratory conditions, a steam inhalation can be an excellent way to influence our mood at the same time. When we are ill with coughs, colds or flu, our mood and energy levels can suffer as much as our airways – so an opportunity to include some mood-enhancing or uplifting oils seems too good to miss. Usually, a bowl of pre-boiled water is placed into a heat proof bowl with three or four drops of essential oil. Then a towel is placed over both client/ patient and bowl, and they are left to inhale through the nose and mouth, taking regular breaks. Less is more here. Since we are inhaling the vapour at a close range, there is a chance that the eyes or mucous membranes of the respiratory tract could become irritated. Make sure to take regular breaks, and only use a minimal amount of oil. Use heat proof gloves when handling hot bowls of water, and take care not to scald yourself on the hot steam.

SPRAYS

A spray makes a lovely way to fragrance a room without the need for electronic devices or heat. Sprays can be home-made or bought pre-blended from aromatherapy suppliers. Generally these products are not designed to be applied to the skin since they usually contain ethanol which can be drying or an irritant.[142] I have made sprays to help clients feel more energised, calm, or to help them prepare for sleep.

PHYSICAL BENEFITS OF AROMATHERAPY

We now know that the emotional effects of aromatherapy are best experienced by inhalation. But what about the physical benefits? Whilst some of the molecules we inhale will of course reach our bloodstream, if we want to have a targeted physical effect on a specific area of the body, there are other methods to consider.

OUR SKIN

In 'Aromatics in Aromatherapy' we explored how the small molecular size of most essential oil compounds makes them volatile, and allows them to evaporate easily. but this is not the only benefit to being so small – their size means that they can easily pass through the tiniest openings in the skin, and have an effect on a localised or systemic (whole-body) level. But size is only half the equation. In 'The Essence of a Plant?' we looked at how essential oils tend to be more fat-soluble due to the lipophilic molecules they contain. This affinity for fat means that these tiny, fat-soluble essential oil molecules can pass into the bloodstream via absorption through our sebaceous ducts, hair follicles and the *stratum corneum* or outer layer of our skin.[143] There are a number of ways we can apply essential oils to our skin, for use in the treatment of muscular, skin, or joint conditions, or as part of a holistic aromatherapy massage treatment.

BALMS AND SALVES

A balm or salve is an oil-based product that usually contains a blend of carrier oils and/or waxes which are non-volatile, or 'fixed', as well as herbal extracts and essential oils, which are usually the primary therapeutic ingredients. Aromatic balms and salves can be used for topical application to sprains, strains, bruises and inflamed joints. No water is used in balms and salves, and as such, they can keep for a long time if stored correctly. We'll explore various carrier oils and understand how they are therapeutic in their own right later in this book.

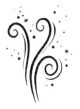

OILS

A blend of carrier and essential oils is a versatile and enjoyable way of applying aromatherapy to the skin. Essential oils are diluted to a safe concentration (usually around 2%) in a carrier oil, and blended to create a therapeutic oil that can be used as part of a massage treatment, or added to a bath.

CREAMS

A blend of water-based products and oils or waxes, a therapeutic cream is ideal for cooling[144] and calming irritating, inflamed skin conditions, such as eczema, where oils or balms, which are considered more energetically 'heating' from a Traditional Western Medicine standpoint, may not be suitable. Creams can also be used daily as part of a skincare regime, but the formulation strength (the dilution of essential oils) should be adjusted accordingly – there is a difference between a concentrated 4% cream for short-term use in acute injuries, and a gentle 1% face cream which can be used on a daily basis.

Safety Notes

You will notice that in the details below, I make reference to a number of percentages and dilutions – don't worry too much if you don't know what these mean yet, since more information about blending and diluting appropriately and safely is given in the recipes and activities throughout the book, as well as in Chapter 7.

COMPRESSES

A compress can be made by soaking a flannel, bandage or cloth in cold or hot water, depending on the desired result. Wring it out, then apply a little of a strong blend of carrier and essential oils (up to 4 or 5%) to the affected area, massaging in gently and then applying the cloth, holding it in place or wrapping it loosely to secure it. Leave this for 30 minutes to an hour at a time, checking occasionally and repeating once or twice a day.

BATHS

An extremely therapeutic full-body, multi sensory experience, and my personal favourite. You can exercise your creative muscles with baths, integrating ritual, herbs, candles, crystals and minerals into the process. But in terms of aromatherapy, blending essential oils with a carrier and adding them to a warm bath will not only improve the skin's absorption of the oils, it will increase the rate of evaporation, so be sure to get in the bath as soon as you add the oil mix!

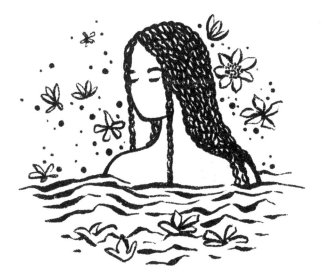

Factors Affecting Absorption

OCCLUSION

Occlusion, or covering an area, as with an aromatherapy compress, speeds up the rate of absorption of the therapeutic blend,[145] which can be useful if fast action is needed, for example on a headache or sprained ankle. Wrapping the area in a towel or cloth following application can help to speed up the healing process. Some therapists use plastic wrap but I prefer a warm, damp cotton cloth instead, to avoid the use of single-use plastic.

TEMPERATURE

Heat is also a factor that speeds up absorption,[146] so warming oil blends prior to application can enhance the effect of topical blends. Alternatively, applying oil during or after a warm bath will dilate the pores in the skin and increase blood flow to the surface, increasing absorption.

SURFACE AREA

Broadly speaking, the more of the area of skin that the blend is applied to, the more therapeutic product will be absorbed.[147] However, it wouldn't necessarily be appropriate to apply a full body massage oil for acute joint pain so it is important to consider the most appropriate application for the issue you want to treat.

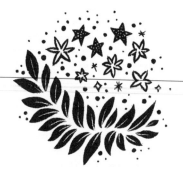

LENGTH OF TIME

The longer you leave the blend in contact with the skin, the more therapeutic product will be absorbed.[148] You may wish to consider leaving an oil blend or cream to absorb following application, or applying an ointment to the affected area multiple times in a day to increase exposure time.

SKIN CONDITION OR TYPE

Dry, cracked or damaged skin may increase dermal absorption of essential oils,[149] but this can be unpredictable and if the skin is damaged, the product could cause irritation so care should be exercised and a lower dilution (1%) should be used in this case. Elderly people and children typically have thinner skin, so a weaker dilution should be used for them (see Safety Notes below).

TYPES OF CARRIER OILS

Carrier oils have varying viscosities[150] and rates of absorption,[151] so depending on which carrier you choose, you may find that some blends absorb more readily than others.

Safety Notes

Great care should be exercised when using essential oils, which should never be ingested, applied undiluted on the skin, or used on children and babies or during pregnancy unless under guidance of a qualified professional. More information on using essential oils safely is available in Chapter 7, and you will find a guide to safe blending ratios in Chapter 4.

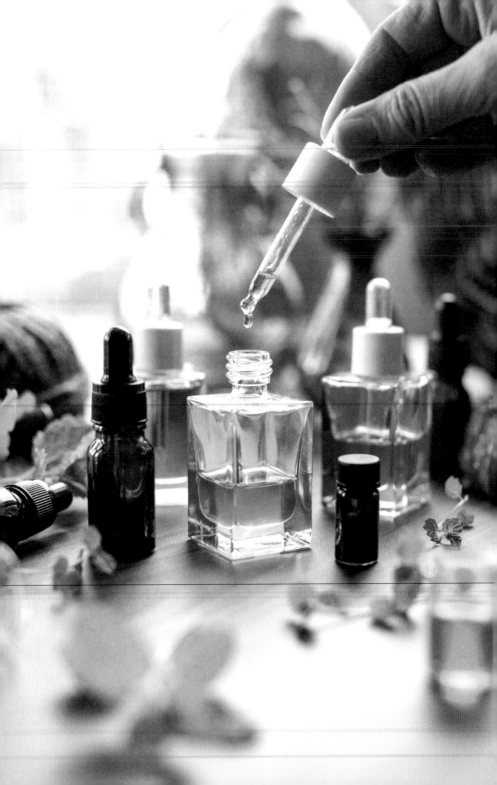

CHAPTER 4
Blending: an Art and a Science

" Nothing is more memorable than a smell.
One scent can be unexpected, momentary and
fleeting, yet conjure up a childhood summer
beside a lake in the mountains." Diane Ackerman[152]

Blending essential oils well is one of the most important skills that an aromatherapist can develop. Learning to blend effectively requires some key ingredients. Firstly, it requires an understanding of what the disease or imbalance is that needs to be addressed. This is fundamental and should inform any therapeutic blend, whether for inhalation or topical application. Secondly, knowledge of the qualities and characteristics, both physical and energetic, of each oil in the aromatherapist's toolkit will mean that oils can be judiciously selected to produce the most effective treatment for the person in question. Interestingly, and perhaps most importantly, two people with a seemingly similar imbalance may leave my treatment room with two very different blends, as not only does the choice of oils matter, but choosing the right ones for the person and their own characteristics and energetic disposition is also important to consider.

The Synergy of Blending

Over time, you'll develop an understanding of the synergies between the oils themselves, and how the plants' various medicinal properties and actions can actually work together to enhance each other, creating a treatment blend that is more than just the sum of its parts. Sajah Popham's book, *Evolutionary Herbalism*, contains an excellent section on herbal synergy for those keen to read more on this topic.[153] Learning how to gain a combined understanding of the various qualities of human, plant and disease takes time and patience to develop, and I'm certainly still learning this every day in my own treatment room and practice. You can read more about herbal energetics in the pull-out section above.

Dilution Ratios

Another important element of blending is safety and dilution ratios. If you are planning to use a blend topically, i.e. on the skin, it's important to blend the essential oils with a carrier oil. For the purposes of massage oil blends, or general-purpose blends for the skin such as body oils or lotions, this is usually at a ratio of 2%. This equates to approximately six drops of essential oil for 10ml of carrier oil, 12 drops for 20ml, and 18 drops for 30ml (1fl oz). The recipes and activities you'll find in this book all state the percentages and number of drops to use, to guide you if you're new to blending. You can also find a useful chart on the Tisserand Institute website.[154]

Blending for Therapeutic Effect

We already know that aromatherapy can have effects on body, mind and soul when it is administered in different ways. But what about the oils themselves? How do we choose which ones to include in a blend, and which ones to leave out, depending on the effect we want to create? There is no exact formula – since all people are unique, so their treatment will be – but below are some guidelines and principles which I hope will help you to begin blending and build confidence as you go. In Chapter 6 you'll find profiles of key essential oils that have been specially selected for their wide range of therapeutic applications, multifunctionality and relative safety and ease of use. I've also included some recipes that will help you understand how they work and how they might be incorporated into different blends.

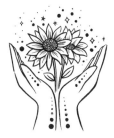

PSYCHO-EMOTIONAL

I tend to find that using the humoral, elemental and energetics-based approaches found in systems of traditional medicine lend themselves particularly well to selecting oils for emotional wellbeing. As such, I use a combination of Ayurveda, Traditional Chinese Medicine and Traditional Western Medicine energetics to decide which ones to use for a particular emotional imbalance. However, as we have seen, there is plenty of research available that supports the use of essential oils for psychological treatment such as anxiety and depression, so I always use this approach alongside my knowledge of the chemistry and pharmacological action of the oils, and use research to understand which oils have sedative, calming or nervine effects, if I'm treating someone who is experiencing insomnia, for example.

PHYSICAL

Essential oils are packed with molecules with a range of medicinal actions, including anti-inflammatory, antiviral, antibacterial, antispasmodic and analgesic, to name just a few. When choosing oils to induce a physical effect, in acute conditions, it is important to consider the primary need, and try to keep the blend focused on that as much as possible. For example, a sprained ankle would likely need anti-inflammatory and analgesic effects in the first instance, so the oils I would choose would be centred around these actions. For more chronic physical conditions, a combination of emotional and physical properties may be more appropriate, since longer-term conditions often come accompanied by complicated, evolving feelings and states of being on both physical and psycho-emotional levels.

AESTHETIC OR PERSONALITY-BASED

Whilst not strictly aromatherapy, blending for aesthetic purposes (i.e. the pure enjoyment of a particular blend) or to match one's personality is arguably therapeutic in its own right. I love to experiment with natural perfumery blends, and even teach a workshop on this very topic. It is really exciting when I see participants thinking outside the box and coming up with innovative or unusual blends. Working in this way from time to time also challenges me to think in a different way from my usually therapeutic perspective. Perfumery is a whole other topic in itself, but the general rule for blending the various 'notes' is the 30-50-20 ratio: 30% of the blend should be your 'top note' oil, so typically lighter, more volatile oils such as citrus and lighter florals. 50% should be your 'mid note' which forms the heart of the blend; these are typically herbaceous or heavier floral scents. Then the last 20% should be your 'base note', which 'fixes' the blend, adding depth and length. Of course, these rules are merely there for guidance and can be broken at will once you get to grips with them. Do be mindful of safety and any contraindications though, and make sure you're using oils appropriately. Even when not intended for therapeutic use, these are still powerful substances and can illicit undesired effects if you're not careful! If you prefer to create a blend that's based on your own aroma personality profile, you might want to refer to Valerie Ann Worwood's nine essential-oil-personality groups for inspiration, which were discussed in Chapter 3.

CREATING SPACE FOR IMAGINATION

My last tip for successful blending is to be playful and experiment. Historically, I was always a diehard citrus fan – but I found that playing around with my blends and adding some depth through combining zesty citrus with floral, woody or spicy notes made for some really intriguing blends. It can be difficult to know where to begin, so some of my workshop participants find it helpful to start with an idea of a place, feeling, state of being or an image in mind, to guide them in choosing their oils. For example, I've known people to create blends based on the feeling they wish to create to help them meditate, sleep, or to relax and bring them into the present when stressed. Images and memories such as the scent of jasmine on the breeze during a warm summer night, or even the depth and serenity of a pine forest have been invoked by students to guide the blending practice. Creating the space for this imaginative approach to arise feels important, so I'd recommend finding a clean, quiet space where you can focus, feel calm, tune in to your breathing and let your imagination gently take hold. For me, this often means sitting in my garden or with a window open so I can hear the world outside, smell the air and feel a breeze. I particularly enjoy the sound of rainfall, seeing plants growing and changing in the garden and hearing birdsong. Making the whole process multi-sensory in this way means I am more connected to the life going on around me, feel connected to the plants that provided the oils I'm using, and often come up with more interesting, effective blends as a result. Sometimes, blends are inspired by my surroundings, which can lead me on a sensory journey through the oils. This is quite interesting when it comes to perfumery blending; imagination coupled with your environment can help create the magic that conjures a mood, feeling, memory or experience through scent.

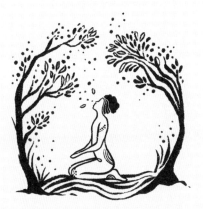

How To Blend

Generally speaking, I advise my workshop participants to begin by blending just three oils, especially if they are new to aromatherapy. This helps keep things simple and allows them to discern between the various aromas without overcomplicating their blend. I advise them to inhale each oil in turn, on a fragrance test strip, as they get to know each one in its own right. Then, they test their combinations by holding the strips together, inhaling with each new addition. This allows them to make sure the blend is right before making up the final product in their carrier oil or diffuser. Now might be a good time to practice this technique yourself before we dive deeper into some of the other ways we can get in touch with aromatic plants and harness their healing potential.

CARRIER OILS

There is a wide range of base (carrier) oils to which we add essential oils in order to dilute them, but these have therapeutic properties in their own right. Here are several examples of carrier oils you may wish to choose from when creating your blends and recipes.

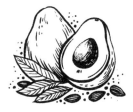

AVOCADO (Persea americana) OIL

Excellent skin penetrator, more so than other carrier oils as the absorption is slower due to the oil's higher viscosity (thickness).[155] It is emollient (softening) and anti-inflammatory.[156]

There are no known contraindications associated with avocado oil, but it's always a good idea to do a patch test to rule out allergies before use.[157]

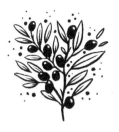

OLIVE (*Olea europaea*) OIL

Antioxidant (rich in vitamin E), anti-inflammatory, anti-microbial, and contains the emollient (skin softener) squalene.[158]

Olive oil is generally safe with a low potential for irritating the skin,[159] however some studies show it can exacerbate atopic dermatitis (eczema).[160] It's always a good idea to do a patch test to rule out allergies before use.

SWEET ALMOND (*Prunus amygdalus* var. *dulcis*) OIL

An excellent emollient (skin softener), this oil makes a good all-purpose massage or base oil, as it is light and hardly has any fragrance.[161]

This oil is non-irritant and safe for topical use,[162] but check for nut and seed allergies before use.

COCONUT (*Cocos nucifera*) OIL

Rich in medium-chain fatty acids.[163] Very light in texture but not quickly absorbed by skin,[164] this makes an excellent massage oil, since fast absorption is undesirable in this case. It is normally solid at room temperature in the UK so will likely need gentle heating before it can be combined with other ingredients. Check for nut or seed allergies before use.

Safe for topical use.[165] However, coconut oil is high in saturated fats,[166] hence it's not easily absorbed by the skin, so may be comedogenic (cause blackheads or acne by blocking pores) for some people.

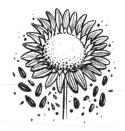

SUNFLOWER (*Helianthus annuus*) OIL

This oil contains up to 60% linoleic acid, which is beneficial for the skin, since it helps our skin to make its own fats which help to repair and smooth the skin.

Generally considered safe and non-irritant.[167] Those with nut or seed allergies should check before using.

INFUSED OILS

Infused oils are carrier oils such as olive or avocado which have been infused with a medicinal herb to enhance its therapeutic effect. Common examples of these are calendula-infused or St. John's wort-infused oils. You might like to experiment with using infused oils once you develop confidence with blending, since they can be a lovely way to add an extra dimension of healing to your recipes and blends.

ST. JOHN'S WORT (*Hypericum perforatum*) INFUSED OIL

St. John's wort is an anti-inflammatory herb, so this oil makes a great topical infused oil for treating burns, reddened skin and bruises; it helps heal sores and ulcers and is calming for neuralgia and sciatica (inflamed nerves).[168]

While St John's wort-infused oil is for topical use only in this book, it is important to note that this herb is commonly taken internally for treating depression. When taken orally St. John's wort can cause interactions with commonly used medications because of how it gets broken down by the liver. When taken internally, this herb can interact with medication in different ways. It can make some drugs less effective while making the effect of others stronger. It should be avoided in pregnancy. It can also increase skin's sensitivity to sunlight, so care should be taken not to expose skin to UV light after topical application.[169] If you're not sure if this oil is suitable for you, please consult a qualified medical herbalist before using it, and don't consume the herb unless under the guidance of a qualified medical herbalist.

POT MARIGOLD, OR CALENDULA
(*Calendula officinalis*) INFUSED OIL

As an external/topical (applied to skin) herbal remedy, calendula is antimicrobial, tissue-healing, antifungal, antiseptic and anti-inflammatory, and is commonly used in the treatment of disorders including dermatitis, broken or varicose veins, or to help heal abrasions (such as burns or cuts) to the skin.[170][171]

This infused oil is generally safe but application should be avoided in pregnancy unless under the supervision of a qualified medical herbalist.[172]

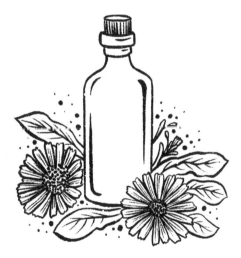

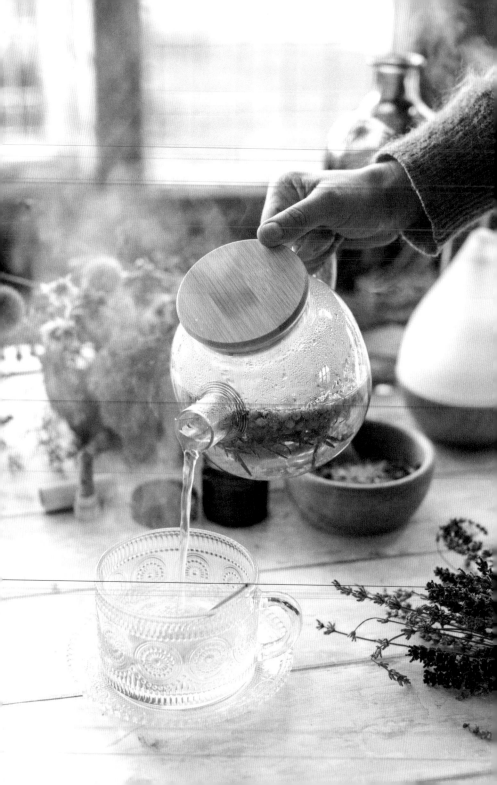

CHAPTER 5

Connecting with Aromatic Plants

" Not knowing the name of the tree, I stood in the flood of its sweet scent." Matsuo Bashō[173]

While we have touched on how to connect with essential oils during the blending process, for me a key part of the healing power of scent is remembering where these incredible essential oils come from in the first place, and appreciating and respecting this. In light of this, here are my three Os – Observation, Olfaction and Organoleptics – three ways for you to connect with the plants that gift us their medicine, and will hopefully enable you to learn about them in a holistic way. The exercises in this chapter are very much led by the plants and don't require too much prior knowledge of botany, herbal medicine or aromatherapy, aside from ensuring that you have correctly identified any plants you plan to interact with, for safety reasons.

Safety Notes

For the activities that follow, if you're not 100% sure of a plant's identification don't use it – misidentification can lead to serious poisoning, and some plants look very similar! Please don't pick the plants for the observation exercise; and only harvest what you need from a clean, plentiful place for the olfaction and organoleptics exercises. See the safe plant finding advice in Chapter 7.

Observation

Observation
noun. /ɒlˈfæk.ʃən/
The action of observing, watching or noticing.[174]

It's amazing what we can find simply by paying attention to what is going on under and around our feet. In my first role at the Royal Botanic Gardens, Kew, I worked on a project called Grow Wild, which is an outreach programme designed to help more people engage with UK-native plants and fungi. During the summer of 2020, I ran a campaign on social media asking the community to send in photos of their observations of wildflowers growing in unlikely places whilst out on their daily walks or exercise. It was incredible to see that so many of these resilient plants popped up in pavement cracks in the most inhospitable of environments, thriving against the odds, providing bursts of colour and life in grey city streets, and a vital food source for pollinators in otherwise pretty undiverse urban landscapes. These incredible plants are still largely unnoticed by society in the main, and considered weeds by most. But what if we paid more attention to them? What might they teach us about themselves, their properties, and their environment? What might we learn about ourselves by reflecting on their growing habits, life cycles, and properties?

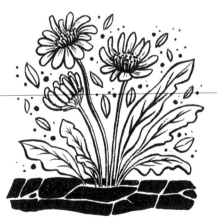

ACTIVITY: GETTING IN TOUCH
WITH AROMATIC PLANTS

Botanists use the power of close observation to tell them important characteristics and distinctions between different plant species in order to classify, identify and understand them on a scientific level. But we can borrow some of these approaches and adapt them in different ways to learn about essential-oil producing plants from many angles. Aromatic, medicinal plants such as *Rosa canina* (dog rose), *Melissa officinalis* (lemon balm), *Mentha × piperita* (peppermint), *Matricaria chamomilla*, *Chamamelum nobile* (German and Roman chamomile) and *Lavandula angustifolia* (lavender) are all grown fairly commonly in gardens, parks and even escape into streets, cycle paths or hedgerows and will all work well for this activity.

I invite you to find an aromatic plant that you can correctly identify in a public green space or street near you. Do not pick or uproot it. You may wish to bring a small sketchbook and pencils, some paints, or some other means to record your thoughts. There is no right or wrong way to approach the exercise; how you record your findings is up to you. Simply observe the plant, and record, draw, paint or write what you notice about it.

SOME POINTS TO CONSIDER

› Look at the plant. How does it make you feel?

› Does it seem to have a particular character, energy or quality?

› Pay particular attention to the plant's features, including its leaves, stems, flowers and colours. What do you notice about them?

› Does the plant live in a particular habitat? Is it wet, dry, shaded or sunny? Does it grow alongside any other plant species?

› What does the plant smell like? Does its aroma conjure up a feeling, memory or sensation?

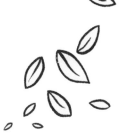

> What colours does it have? What textures?

> Does it attract any pollinators, or other wildlife? Which ones?

> How might its shape, form and growing habits lend themselves to the plant's resilience or survival?

> What time of year is it? What time of day is it? Do you see flowers, leaves or seeds?

> Has the plant overcome any challenges to survive? Has it adapted to its situation in any way?

> How is the plant unique?

> Come back in a few weeks and visit the plant. How has it changed?

By using our powers of observation to consider an aromatic plant, we might find that we learn something new about its qualities, character or habits. Maybe these observations could give you a clue as to some of its energetic or medicinal qualities? If you would like to dive deeper into the world of plant-led learning, Nathaniel Hughes and Fiona Owens' book, *Weeds in the Heart*, is a beautiful guide to getting to know some common medicinal and aromatic plants in an intuitive way.

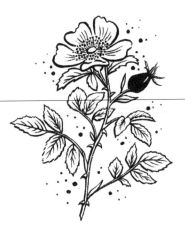

Nature and Wellbeing

GREEN SOCIAL PRESCRIBING

An increasing number of studies show that spending more time in green spaces can have a positive impact on our mental health and wellbeing.[175] 'Green social prescribing' in particular is a growing area within healthcare as pilot projects are set up as alternative treatments for a range of mental health conditions, and to improve and enhance social care.[176] Activities available through community projects or charitable initiatives that may connect us to the healing power of scent include community gardening, cookery, fermentation, walking or even forest bathing.

SENSORY GARDENS

Sensory gardens are usually cultivated green spaces specifically designed with our senses in mind – smell in particular, since aroma is so important in plant reproduction and survival, attracting pollinators and, yes, humans. These gardens lead us on a journey through textured, colourful and scented herbs that are a feast for the eyes and interesting to the touch. But wandering through a sensory garden really gives us the opportunity to 'stop and smell the roses', inhaling their soothing volatile oils whilst soaking in the biodiversity, beauty and variety that surrounds us.

SHINRIN-YOKU

The Japanese practice of forest bathing is brilliant as it doesn't require anything of the participant other than simply taking in the atmosphere of the forest through all the senses. It's therefore relatively accessible, and can be enjoyed sitting, standing, lying down or while walking. If you don't have access to large forests, a local green space such as a park still provides a multi-sensory experience that can enhance wellbeing. Salvatore Battaglia, a renowned aromatherapist, argues that humans are drawn to essential oils since we have an inherent connection to the natural world, and working with essential oils (responsibly and sparingly, I would add) is a way to summon and strengthen that connection.[177] It is my hope, and that of research scientists[178] and global institutions like the UN,[179] that by strengthening this bond through exploring more ways to reconnect with nature, and through education, we can deepen our appreciation of – and our resolve to protect – the natural world of which we are an intrinsic part.

Olfaction

Olfaction
noun. UK /ɒlˈfæk.ʃən/
The action of smelling; the capacity for smelling; the sense of smell.[180]

In Chapter 1 we looked at our sense of smell, its mysteries, complexities, its chemistry and biology. Putting the science to one side, though, smell provides an excellent medium through which to get to know our healing scented plants and their oils. In the observation exercise, we explored how using multiple senses can teach us about an aromatic plant and its properties. But isolating just one of our senses, in this case the sense of smell, can allow us to go deeper into the qualities, properties and feelings associated with each essential oil. In my workshops, we often participate in collective 'blind' aroma sampling exercises, where we spend some time experiencing the oil on an individual level, before coming together to share our experiences with the group. The exercise below is an adapted version of this, which also allows you to record your experiences of each oil you inhale. I recommend coming back and experiencing the same oil multiple times throughout the year, since how you experience a particular aroma may well change over time, depending on the day, hormone levels, what is going on in your life, or the time of year. You can also do this exercise in small groups, taking it in turns to be the facilitator, and hand around the oils, so everyone can experience an oil without knowing what it is first. I find this way of working best, since knowing the plant can often colour our interpretations. While I usually carry out this activity with essential oils, you can do it with leaves, flowers, roots, bark, seeds, live plants, spices or fruits – providing you know what they are, and that they are safe to use. You could even compare a live plant to its corresponding essential oil and note down the differences you observe.

ACTIVITY: MAKING A SCENT DIARY

In *Fragrance and Wellbeing*, Jennifer Peace Rhind argues that simply by improving and training our olfactory palate, we may experience wellbeing benefits.[181] I have certainly found this to be true in my own practice, and have received wonderful feedback from my workshop participants who have all tried the exercise I will share with you below.

Creating a scent diary is about more than just recording and learning about aromas. It is a way for you to develop your own relationship with the essential oils and other aromas you come across as you go through the world, and record your own, unique experiences, interpretations of and responses to them. I hope that it will enable you to build, over time, your own bank of fragrances that you can draw on to deepen your understanding of aromas, herbs and their effects.

While you may find lots of information in books that detail the therapeutic, energetic and chemical properties of an oil, building your own mini-profiles as part of a scent dictionary will undoubtedly add a unique and subjective element to your learning, and hopefully enrich the experience, so that it becomes a personal practice and wellbeing experience for you, in and of itself.

Now that we've learned how to sample an essential oil, you could begin with this technique before branching out further to explore your environment and all the scents it holds...

YOU WILL NEED

› A small notebook (or A-Z address book if you prefer)

› Pencils or pens

› Scents: perfumes, essential oils, flowers, or the natural environment (see Safety Notes at the beginning of this chapter)

› Aroma sampling stick

› A comfortable and preferably peaceful spot to sit (in nature, a park, indoors or in an urban environment will all work fine)

HOW TO CREATE YOUR SCENT DIARY

There are lots of ways to approach the creation of a scent diary, and the good news is that there is no one right way to do it. Below, I have suggested some approaches and elements for you to consider, but I would encourage you to play around with how you record aromas to discover what works best for you. I'd love to see what ideas you come up with – you can share your creations with me via @amberluna_apothecary.

Using a table

This is a version of a table I use in my aroma workshops so that students can begin to record their own responses to aromas. You may wish to make your own version in your notebook so that you can record your own experiences. The examples below were recorded from an aroma sampling with essential oils, but you could use other scents: found leaves, flowers, and tree bark, or even urban scents as you walk around the city (if you're planning to find plants while out and about see the Safety Notes at the beginning of this chapter).

Aroma/plant/ essential oil name	Lavender essential oil (Lavandula angustifolia)	Bitter orange essential oil (Citrus x aurantium var. amara)
Visualised colour	Pale green, sage green	Yellow, egg yolk
Shapes	Smooth, flowing, wisps of smoke	Sunburst, jagged
Adjectives	Heavy, grounding, thick	Bursting, opening, enlivening, fresh
Temperature	Cooling	Neutral to warm
Dry/moist?	Dry	Moist, fresh
Memory/imagery	Mediterranean hillsides	Holidays by the coast
Where does it 'travel' in my body?	Nose, lungs, chest, head	Head, heart
Feeling	Peace	Joy
Do I like this scent?	Yes	Yes

Journal style

If you prefer, you could take a more prose-based approach to record your experiences. Nature journaling is a technique that sits at the intersection between science, mindfulness and art[182] whereby we note, illustrate and capture our observations from spending time in our natural environment in a journal. A similar approach can be used to document our observations of a certain aroma. You could draw, write, collage, or even add perfumes and essential oil drops to the pages of your journal to create a multi-dimensional, multi-sensory experience.

Herbal monograph style

A herbal monograph is a paper written on a specific herb, including its properties,[183] botany, and medicinal uses, but can even include folklore and is often illustrated. Some of the old herbals from the 17th century onwards have stunningly illustrated examples of medicinal plants.[184] You might want to take inspiration from them, creating your own aromatic monographs. A good, free, online resource to use for inspiration is Mrs Grieve's *A Modern Herbal*,[185] originally published in 1931 but now digitised and available for free, online. Bear in mind that some of the information in the *Herbal* is now out of date, so this shouldn't be used as an up-to-date medicinal herb guide. I recommend it here so you can explore what sorts of information to include in your scent diary, and see the images that are included.

A-Z style

You could even make shorter entries in an A-Z address book, if you prefer to build a scent diary more quickly. Small address books are usually cheap, easy to source and convenient to take with you should you wish to make entries on your travels. Sometimes the magic of scent can capture us at the strangest moments – so this is a good option if you don't want to miss anything!

Language, Mindfulness and the Art of Capturing Scent

As we've previously explored, in describing aromas, we are heavily reliant on language – which is so often insufficient to communicate all of the symbolic nuances that aroma can evoke.[186] By becoming playful and creative with the words you use to describe an aroma, you might start to develop and enrich your olfactory vocabulary and discover a whole new language with which to interpret and describe the world around you. Pause, take a deep breath as you inhale, and for each new scent consider what you think, feel, and experience as you inhale. Pay attention at each moment, notice how the aromas change in quality, texture and strength. Once you have been sitting with your plant or scent, thank it in your own way, and pause to jot down your notes or drawings.

Organoleptics

Organoleptic
adj. UK /ɔːˌganə(ʊ)ˈlɛptɪk/
Of, relating to, or involving the use of sense organs or senses, esp. of smell and taste.[189]

Organoleptic tasting or testing, in the context of aromatherapy and herbalism, means using our sensory abilities, particularly our senses of smell and taste, to understand aromatic herbs' characters, qualities and properties. It is a technique I continue to use throughout my aromatherapy practice and herbalism training, and has been well understood by practitioners throughout the ages to help them develop a more intuitive and sensory understanding of the plants they work with. It has some crossovers with the observation exercise we practiced previously, although this one focuses more on taste and smell. I have been taught – and found it to be true – that this process is best conducted without knowing what the herb is in advance, so if you can recruit a friend to help prepare the herbs or oils without revealing which herb is being presented, it can be a brilliant way to remove the possibility of bias in your interpretations and experiences, based on your previous knowledge of the herbs.

During an organoleptic herb experience, a hot infusion (herbs steeped and covered in near-boiling water for about ten minutes) can be prepared using a singular, aromatic, medicinal plant, either fresh or dried. With this method, you'll be inhaling the volatile aromatic oils as the hot water releases them from the plant, tasting the water-soluble compounds, and examining the colours and textures of the plant through looking and feeling the infusion in your mouth.

Safety Notes

This way of ingesting essential oils, in a fresh or dried herb infusion, is safe since you'll be taking in very low quantities. I have also included a scent-only version of the following exercise, so that you can practice aroma sampling with essential oils on fragrance sticks, but note that these highly-concentrated extracts are not safe to ingest in an undiluted form (see Chapter 7).

ACTIVITY: HERB TASTING EXERCISE

Tasting a herb without knowing what it is will free you of all preconceptions –try it in this exercise.

YOU WILL NEED

> 1-2 tsp of dried (or a small handful of fresh) aromatic herbs (see Safety Notes at the beginning of this chapter). Suggested options if you're new to aromatic herbs include German chamomile, lemon balm, rose or peppermint

> A friend to help, if you are going to do a 'blind' tasting

> Filtered, pre-boiled water, at approx 85-90°C (185-195°F). If you don't have a thermometer, simply boil the water and leave it to cool for a few minutes before pouring.

> A teacup

> A filter or tea strainer that will fit into the teacup

> Something to cover the cup with, like a small dish or jar lid

> A notebook or sketchbook

> Pens or pencils

METHOD

1 Add your herb to the filter or strainer and place it in the cup.

2 Add around 200-250ml (6½-8½floz) of the pre-boiled water to the herb, depending on the size of your teacup

3 Inhale the aroma as the hot water touches the herb, being careful not to scald yourself on the steam.
   > What do you notice about the scent?
   > How does the herb's colour, texture or appearance change as the hot water touches it?
   > Write your observations down, draw them, or record them in another way.

4 Once your cup is full, cover and leave for 10 minutes to infuse.

5 Once 10 minutes is up, lift out the strainer and set the infused herb to one side.

6   Find somewhere quiet to sit with your herb, and observe the liquid in the cup.
    › What colours does it have now, after infusing for a while?
    › How is the clarity of the liquid?
    › When you swirl it around the cup, does it change?
    › Does the infusion have a particular texture?

7   Now, bring the cup close to your face. Inhale.
    › Does this herb have an aroma after it has been infused?
    › How has the initial aroma changed from pre- to post-infusion?
    › Does the aroma change from the beginning, through
      the middle and to the end of the inhalation?
    › Does it conjure any images, memories, textures or feelings?
    › Again, record your observations.

8   Now it's time to taste. Make sure that the infusion has cooled enough, then close
    your eyes and take a sip. Hold the liquid in your mouth for a few moments, and
    swirl it around if you like. Then swallow.
    › What do you notice about the flavour? Does it change over time?
    › Does the infusion have a texture or 'mouthfeel'?
    › Which areas of your tongue 'light up' as you taste?
      Bitter, sweet, umami, salty or sour?
    › Does the infusion leave an aftertaste? What is it like?
    › As you drink, you can repeat steps 6 to 8 as many times as you like.

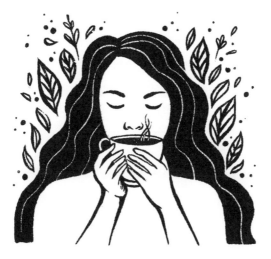

9 Sit quietly for a few moments once you've finished your cup. I find it helps to keep my eyes closed so I can tune in to how I feel. You may like to take notice of any changes to how you feel, physically, emotionally, mentally or energetically.

› Does the herb appear to 'travel' anywhere in your body?
› Do you feel a change in your body's temperature?
› How does your mood feel now compared to before you drank the infusion? Are there any emotions that arise?
› Do you feel a connection to the herb you've just tried?
› What might the ways you now feel tell you about this herb's properties?
› Do you like this herb?
› Does this herb have a personality? This may be a word, quality or feeling.

Again, record your findings. This exercise is sensory and intuitive and therefore there are no wrong answers, since your responses to the herb are yours alone and totally subjective! It's common for a group of people to have quite different responses to individual herbs, so don't worry if your perceptions and experiences don't match up with what you've read or heard about this herb previously. I'd suggest practicing this technique with one herb several times over a few months, so you can see how your own perceptions may change over time, too. I have found this exercise to be a great way to get to know an aromatic plant on an individual level and begin to build a relationship with it as a whole plant, and not just with the essential oil it produces, although it is also very helpful to do this exercise with only your sense of smell, comparing the fresh herb, dried herb and essential oils to each other, noting the differences between them, and the qualities of each.

ACTIVITY: AROMA SAMPLING EXERCISE

Here is a version of the organoleptic activity using only scent. This exercise will allow you to deepen your relationship with single aromas and come to understand their complexity and character.

YOU WILL NEED

› Aromatic herbs (see Safety Notes at the beginning of this chapter). I suggest working with one plant at a time, to include:

› The fresh herb (small handful of the herb, fruit or a live plant in a pot will all work)

› The dried herb (1-2 tsp)

› The essential oil (bottle)

› Fragrance sticks for sampling

the essential oils. Use compostable cotton buds if you can't get hold of these.

› A friend, if doing a 'blind' aroma sampling

› Small bowl for the dried herb

› A notebook or sketchbook

› Pens or pencils

METHOD

1 Find a quiet space with a table.

2 Place your fresh plant on the table, along with some of the dried herb in a bowl, and a fragrance stick with a couple of drops of your chosen essential oil. If you are doing a 'blind' aroma sampling, then close your eyes and ask your friend to present them to you one by one, stating whether fresh, dried, or essential oil.

3   Crush a little of the fresh herb in your hand to release the essential oils. Then do the same for the dried herb if possible. This is unnecessary for the fragrance stick with essential oils, since the oil has already been 'released' from the plant through distillation.

> For each version of the herb, think about the following:
> How long does it take for the aroma to reach your nose?
> What does the aroma remind you of? Does it conjure any memories?
> Does the aroma feel hot, cold, moist, dry, light or heavy?
> Does it smell earthy, flowery, fruity, herbal, spicy, grassy or resinous? Are there any other words you'd use to describe the aroma?
> Are there any textures or images you associate with this aroma?
> Do you like the aroma?
> What personality does the herb have? Does it have a particular quality?
> How do you feel when you inhale its aroma? Does this differ depending on whether it is fresh, dried, or in essential oil form?
> Does the aroma change over time? Perhaps come back to the herb an hour later and smell it again.
> How do the three forms of the herb compare to one another?

Record your findings. You might wish to repeat the exercise with more individual herbs, before then selecting two or more plants to compare to one another. If you do this, I'd suggest picking either two essential oils, or two fresh or dried plants, and comparing them instead of working on all three forms of the herb. You might find that you are better able to draw comparisons between them.

Tip: You might find it useful to add some of your experiences from these organoleptic exercises to your scent diary, so you can refer to them at a later date.

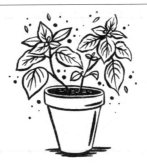

Infusion Recipe

Once you've familiarised yourself with the process of organoleptic tasting and smelling, you might want to branch out and make some of your own aromatic herb infusion blends. Below, you'll find my recipe for an aromatic herbal infusion blend that I love to make as a soothing, cleansing drink that while calming, is non-drowsy so can be drunk at any time of day. It works well drunk hot, or as a cooled iced tea in hot weather.

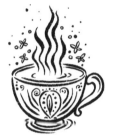

Nurture, Calm and Cleanse Tea

This tea contains five aromatic herbs as well as one non-aromatic but very soothing herb, marshmallow. Below, I have included some information on calendula and marshmallow, neither of which are very aromatic and don't yield essential oils, but are nonetheless therapeutic in their own right. You can find information on each of the other aromatic herbs' actions, uses, energetic qualities, symbolism and aromas in the plant profile pages in Chapter 6.

Safety Notes: While all the herbs in this recipe have been chosen for their relative safety as well as their medicinal properties, before you ingest anything please make sure you read the advice in Chapter 7 and see the warnings about using certain substances while pregnant or breastfeeding.

- Large mixing bowl (metal, ceramic or glass)

- Scales and a small bowl for weighing each herb

- Tongs or a wooden spoon

- Wide-neck funnel (not essential, but makes life easier!)

- 5g (³⁄₁₆oz) dried pot marigold or calendula (*Calendula officinalis*) flowers

- 5g (³⁄₁₆oz) dried rose (*Rosa × damascena*) flowers

- 15g dried bitter orange (*Citrus × aurantium*) peel

- 10g (⅓oz) dried marshmallow (*Althaea officinalis*) root

- 5g (³⁄₁₆oz) dried lemon balm (*Melissa officinalis*) leaves

- 10g (⅓oz) dried German chamomile (*Matricaria chamomilla*) flowers

- Sealable bag or jar to store the herb blend

- Label and pen

- Makes 50g (1³⁄₄oz) total, but you can make larger quantities if you like it!

Note: If you don't have space to grow and dry your own herbs, then you can buy these as dried herbs from many online retailers or whole food shops. I recommend sourcing organic herbs wherever possible.

Safety Notes

Calendula oil is safe for use externally but internal use of the herb should be avoided in pregnancy.

Lemon balm essential oil (Melissa) should be used at a dilution of 1% or less for topical (skin preparations. Lemon balm essential oil should not be used during pregnancy or if breastfeeding.

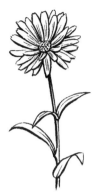

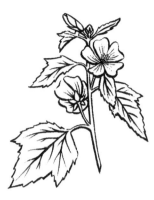

POT MARIGOLD, OR CALENDULA
(*Calendula officinalis*)
Marigold is a brilliant, uplifting, cleansing herb, which has a wide range of health-supporting actions.

Actions
Antimicrobial, tissue-healing, antifungal, antiseptic, anti-inflammatory.[190]

Used for
Treatment of gastrointestinal inflammation, fevers, chronic infections and for clearing lymphatic congestion.[191]

Energetics and symbolism
A sunshine loving plant, this herb gets its name from the word 'calendar', and blooms pretty much all year round. It is considered hot, dry, and astringent in Traditional Western Medicine.[192]

Scent
Resinous, sharp, sweet, joyful.

MARSHMALLOW
(*Althaea officinalis*)
Marshmallow is a soothing, calming and moistening herb with a softening action.

Actions
Anti-inflammatory, antioxidant,[193] demulcent (soothing to mucous membranes; creates a protective barrier).[194]

Used for
Treatment of irritated mucous membranes and to support tissue regeneration,[195] for example in the gastrointestinal tract.

Energetics and symbolism
Energetically cool and moist.[196] Considered a lunar herb that is both nourishing and softening; used for those who are 'stuck' or 'hardened' emotionally.[197]

Scent
sweet, woody, mild, vanilla-like, gentle.

METHOD

1   Make sure all the ingredients are of a similar size. Your herbs should all be roughly the size of most loose teas. If you source your ingredients from a supplier, they will usually come pre-chopped to size, but if you've grown and dried your own, you'll want to cut them up. You can do this with a knife and chopping board or with scissors for some herbs.

2   Weigh out the herbs one by one into the smaller bowl, and then place them in the larger one.

3   When you've finished, combine the herbs using tongs or a wooden spoon. Make sure the herbs are evenly combined

4   Use a wide neck funnel to decant the herbs into your jar or resealable bag.

5   Label with the name of the blend, ingredients, and date.

6   Store well sealed, in a cool, dry place.

7   To make the infusion, use 1-2 heaped tsp per person and steep, covered, in a teapot or cup with a strainer for 10 minutes. Drink hot, or allow to cool, and refrigerate.

Meditation, Ceremony and Ritual

Historically, aromatic substances have been used as an aid to meditation in ceremonial and religious settings in order to help enhance spiritual connection, as an offering, or to purify a space.[198] Across ancient Egypt, Greece and the Middle East, frankincense (*Boswellia spp.*) has been of significant importance in religious settings, and has subsequently been shown by scientific studies to elicit psychoactive (anxiolytic and antidepressant-like) effects in animals, which may partially explain some of this species' long history of spiritual use.[199] It also has the ability to deepen and regulate breathing, which is key to many forms of meditation practice.[200]

Note: At the time of writing, many species in the Boswellia family are now threatened or critically endangered and therefore their essential oils and resins are no longer sustainable to purchase or use.[201]

Other aromatic plant extracts, as we have seen, can also change our mood and state of mind, so conducting spiritual ceremonies or meditating with the help of plant allies can be very powerful, even if conducted in non-religious settings. While frankincense was traditionally used for sacred purposes, it could equally be appreciated for its heady, woody and entrancing aroma during ceremonies.

While in spiritual settings, oils, scented candles and incense are frequently used to create a particular environment or encourage a meditative state,[202] smell alone is rarely the sole focus of a meditation or ceremony.[203] This is perhaps with the exception of the Japanese tradition of Koh-do, or 'the way of incense', which is both an art form and social practice whereby participants, guided by a facilitator and strict etiquette, explore, play with and interpret various aromas, recording and exploring their findings together.[204]

By taking our scent explorations one step further than we did in the aroma sampling exercise, we can deepen our understanding of the aromatic plants we are working with. This can be experienced through giving dedicated time and space to exploring the use of a single essential oil at a time as the central focus of meditation practice.

The following is a meditation designed to be carried out individually or in a group setting. I have led this exercise in various forms with my workshop groups, and it has often yielded complex and interesting results in terms of the emotions, sensations, insights and images that participants discover through the experience. I find it is best experienced with closed eyes, since in this way, participants can lend their attention entirely on the scent of the essential oils, giving them the freedom to explore the responses invoked within them and their immediate space.

ACTIVITY: AROMATIC MEDITATION

Use this activity to explore your responses to your chosen scent at a deeper level.

YOU WILL NEED

> Water

> A chosen aromatic herb (see Safety Notes at the beginning of this chapter) – fresh if possible, or dried. Use both if you have them.

> The essential oil of your chosen herb

> A plate or a piece of fabric in the same colour as your herb (to make a herbal shrine)

> A clean, quiet space to sit – on the floor, a cushion or chair

> An electronic essential oil diffuser or tea-light diffuser

> A tissue or aroma sampling strip

> Stones, flowers, bark or seeds for decoration (optional)

MEDITATION

1   Place the plate or cloth on a table in front of you, or on the floor.

2   Decorate the cloth with your chosen herb at the centre, as well as any other decorations.

3   Add 5-10 drops of essential oil to your diffuser along with some water and light it or turn it on.

4   Add a few drops of essential oil to your tissue or aroma sampling strip, making sure you have this to hand.

5   Sit on your cushion, the floor or your chair in front of your herbal shrine, finding a comfortable position that you can hold for around five minutes.

6   Close your eyes. Take a deep inhalation for four counts, breathing out for six. Try to be present and allow any thoughts to come and go, if you can.

7   Deepen the breath, taking another deep inhalation for four counts, this time breathing out for eight counts, if you can. Repeat this step, feeling the weight of your body wherever you are sitting right now, and feeling the space around you.

8   Now, slowly, and carefully, hold your aroma strip or tissue up to your nose, taking care not to upset your shrine or diffuser.

9   Keeping your eyes closed, take a long, slow, gentle inhalation, holding the tissue or strip about 2cm away from your nose. Focus on how the aroma reaches your nose, enters your body, and how it affects your mind.

10 Repeat this step, this time taking a slightly deeper inhalation. Notice any changes in the quality of the aroma.

Safety Note: stop, take a break, open your eyes and return to normal breathing if you feel light headed or dizzy.

11 Repeat the inhalation exercise a couple more times, each time focusing on the aroma and its qualities and effects.

12 Now, place the aroma strip or tissue to one side, and sit with your eyes closed for a few more minutes, noticing:
    › How your skin feels now. Are there any sensations?
    › How your body feels now. Is it heavy? Light? Is there any movement?
    › How your mind feels now. Do any thoughts, feelings, or insights come?
    › Do you notice any other experiences, images or sensations?

13 When you feel ready, open your eyes slowly, readjusting to the environment around you. If you feel called to, you might want to write down some of your experiences, or sit quietly for a few more moments so that you can let the effects sink in and reflect on them.

You can repeat this exercise daily or weekly over a period of a month or so, in order to deepen your relationship with a particular plant and oil. Otherwise, you might prefer to work with a different plant each week, noticing the variations and similarities between them. This exercise is really a template, and I'd encourage you to adapt it in a way that works for your life.

Just as every aromatic plant is unique, so will everyone's individual experience of the meditation be. If not much comes up for you during the meditation, I would encourage you to come back to it at another time, and repeat the exercise, since even day to day your experience may change quite significantly. Equally, if none of the suggested points to consider (above) chime with you, then feel free to invent your own.

Once you are confident working with one oil at a time, you can begin creating simple diffuser blends to work with during your meditation practice, whether for use as the main focus of an aroma meditation, or to enhance your existing meditation practice. A suggested blend is included below.

Meditation Blend
(for a diffuser or tea light oil burner)

› 3 drops cedarwood atlas (*Cedrus atlantica*) – grounding, calming, centering

› 4 drops bergamot (*Citrus × bergamia*) – uplifting, relaxing, harmonising

› 3 drops pine (*Pinus sylvestris*) – clarifying, awakening, revitalising

METHOD

Fill your diffuser or tea light oil burner with water. On electronic diffusers there is usually a maximum fill mark on the side of the water reservoir. Add the essential oils to the water in the quantities shown above, and replace the lid on your diffuser or light the tea light below its water chamber. If using a tea light burner, make sure it does not burn dry. Now you are ready to meditate!

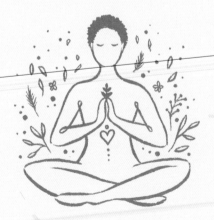

Rest Ritual

Not all rituals need to be spiritual or religious in nature. Some can be simply restful, pleasurable and relaxing, and an antidote to the challenges and demands of a culture that pushes us to always be doing – and being – more. Tricia Hersey, the activist and author of *Rest is Resistance*, is an advocate for rest as a way to 'deprogram, decolonize, and unravel ourselves from the wreckage of capitalism and white supremacy'.[205] I whole-heartedly recommend reading Tricia's work.

This, then, is a ritual both inspired by and celebrating rest. It includes an aromatic and therapeutic oil blend that you can add to a bath, foot soak, or apply post-shower as a nourishing skin or massage oil.

I recommend that you carry out this ritual before bed since the aromatherapy oil blend is designed to help clear the mind, soothe the nervous system and promote good sleep. Better still, make space for a whole day of rest and undertake the ritual in the morning. In the spirit of rest, if planning and carrying out the whole ritual feels like too much, you can simplify it by running a bath or filling a washing up bowl full of warm water and simply adding a handful of fresh mint leaves or some fresh or dried rose petals to the tub. Equally, you could make just the oil blend without the salt soak or herbs.

You will need to prepare a few ingredients and some equipment in advance, so I recommend that you read through the whole activity first to make sure you have what you need before getting started.

PART ONE – PREPARE

Run a bath or fill a small tub with warm water to soak your feet in. If you're opting for a foot soak, place an old towel underneath the tub to avoid splashing the floor. While the tub is filling, prepare your towel for afterwards, and lay out something comfy to wear when you've finished. Prepare a space to rest, with plenty of cushions, blankets, and rugs. You can get really creative here, adding decorations such as objects found in nature, tea lights, scarves, books and other comforts, such as your favourite music, a pad of paper and pencils, and some snacks. If you have access to outside space and it's warm enough, you might like to take a picnic blanket or roll mat and lay it outside in a garden, taking a cool drink with you. Otherwise, make a nest in a quiet room indoors, and brew your favourite cuppa. It's important to make sure you are really comfy, so don't hold back on the cushions and blankets.

Nervous System Nourishing Bath Oil

This bath oil has been designed to nourish and soothe an overstimulated nervous system, so the oils in this blend have been chosen primarily for their calming effects as well as their anti-inflammatory effects for the musculoskeletal system. Please see the plant profile pages for more information on the specific properties of each oil. Use half the recipe for a foot soak or for a post-shower massage oil.

YOU WILL NEED

> 20ml (½fl oz) base (carrier) oil such as sweet almond (*Prunus amygdalus var. dulcis*), coconut (*Cocos nucifera*) or sunflower (*Helianthus annuus*), organic and cold pressed if possible. Otherwise, a good quality cooking oil such as olive oil (*Olea europaea*) will do. See Chapter 7 to check the suitability of your chosen carrier oil.

> Essential oils of German chamomile (*Matricaria chamomilla*), lavender (*Lavandula angustifolia*), and lemon balm (*Melissa officinalis*).

> Medium sized mixing bowl and spoon (not plastic)

> Measuring cup

METHOD

1 Measure out 20ml (½fl oz) of your chosen base oil in the measuring cup.

2 Add up to 12 drops in total of your essential oils; you can play around with the amounts of the individual oils as long as they total no more than 12 drops.

3 Pour the oil blend into the bowl and mix with the spoon. Your oil is now ready to be added to your bath.

Safety Notes

Lemon balm essential oil (Melissa) should be used at a dilution of 1% or less for topical (skin) preparations. Lemon balm essential oil should not be used during pregnancy or if breastfeeding.

Herbal Salt Soak

It is thought that magnesium sulphate may help to increase magnesium levels in the body when absorbed transdermally (via the skin) in a bath, and anecdotal reports cite reduced inflammation, faster muscle recovery, lower stress levels and improved sleep amongst its benefits,[206] but more research is needed in this area. Skip this recipe if you're showering, and use a quarter of the amount of salts for a foot soak!

YOU WILL NEED

> 50g (1¾oz) Himalayan pink salt (or any other sea/rock salt without anti-caking agents or additives)

> 300g (7oz) Epsom salts (magnesium sulphate)

> Handful of fresh peppermint (*Mentha × piperita*) leaves,

and/or fresh or dried rose (*Rosa × damascena*) petals

> Kitchen scales

> Medium sized bowl

> Spoon

METHOD

1 Measure out the salts using the scales and bowl.

2 Chop or tear the fresh herbs and add them, along with any dried petals, to the salts in the bowl.

3 Combine the salt and herb mix with the spoon. Your salt blend is now ready to be added to your bath.

4 If you like, you can add this salt soak mix to the Nervous System Nourishing Bath Oil blend before adding it to a bath, or if you are planning a shower instead, keep them separate so you can massage the oil into your skin afterwards.

Safety Notes

Peppermint (herb or essential oil) should not be used during pregnancy or if breastfeeding.

PART TWO – BATH TIME

Once you've made your herbal salt soak and aromatic oil blend, it's time to put them in the bath. Give them a good stir to ensure the salts dissolve, and the herbs and oils disperse. The steam from the bath will allow the essential oils to slowly evaporate, filling the room's atmosphere with your restful blend. This will also work if you're doing a foot soak. If you're hopping in the shower, skip the salts, and keep the oil blend to massage into your body in circular motions after you've dried off, avoiding the face.

If you like, and it's safe to do so, you could light some unscented tea lights and put them around the bathtub or on a table near your foot bath for added atmosphere. It may be a good idea to take some cold drinking water with you before you get into the bath, in case you overheat.

Once you are in the bath or foot soak, try to focus on relaxing each muscle in your body, one at a time. Take care not to fall asleep, but you can close your eyes if it helps you to tune in to relaxing your body. Then, take some slow, soft inhalations through your nose, letting the different aromatic notes weave their way to you. If you are applying the oil post-shower, you can tune into the aromas as you massage the oil into your skin. As with the aroma sampling exercise and meditation, try to perceive the qualities of the different aromas, notice where they go, how they feel. Take regular sips of cold water or get out if you feel too hot. Soak for around 30 minutes in total.

The hot water from your bath or shower will increase your skin's permeability to the tiny molecules in the essential oils, allowing them and their therapeutic benefits to enter your bloodstream more easily. They will also be inhaled and absorbed via your olfactory system too, so this is a really holistic way to maximise the essential oils' effects on your body and mind.

PART THREE – REST RITUAL

Once you have finished your bath, get out and dry off, then put on your comfy clothes. Now it's time to let the aromatic oils take effect! If you want to continue even further with the aromatic journey, you can use the recipe for the meditation blend from the Aromatic Meditation exercise earlier in this chapter and add it to a diffuser, leaving it on for around 30 minutes. Then, put the kettle on, grab a book, and make yourself comfortable. Make sure you drink plenty of water to stay hydrated, and you might also like to have a light snack.

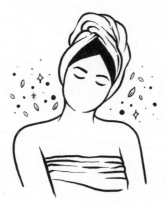

Tune in to your body at regular intervals throughout the day, using some of the reflection points from the Aromatic Meditation activity to help you notice the after-effects of the ritual on your body and mind. Take note of any changes or sensations you experience. You can use this opportunity to do some gentle creative activities like free drawing, sketching, journalling or reading. Alternatively, you might just feel like taking a nap! How you spend the rest of this time is really up to you. I'd encourage you to listen to what your body and mind feel they need, and try to honour that as much as possible. Above all, enjoy the experience!

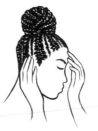

Aromatic Self-care: Prevention and Support for Physical Illness

Whilst aromatherapy can play an important role in supporting our emotional and mental health, there are a number of ways we can harness the healing power of scent for its physical benefits. As well as helping clients to regulate emotions through inhalation and massage, aromatherapists regularly make and supply a wide range of herbal and aromatic products to treat anything from dermatitis to respiratory illness and even poor circulation, since the therapeutic properties of the essential oils, base (carrier) oils or lotions are accessed not just through the nose, but via the skin. This can include oil-based balms, water-based lotions and creams, inhalers, and oil blends. Below, I've included some go-to recipes for treating and preventing a range of common and seasonal complaints. All the recipes have been created using the oils in the plant profiles in this book, so you can see exactly why each ingredient has been included and what effect it has on the body. Give these a go to support your own health throughout the year. I'm always curious to hear about your creations, so feel free to tag me on social media @amberluna_apothecary if you feel called to share.

RESPIRATORY SYSTEM

Some essential oils have a wide range of therapeutic action for our respiratory system. I remember herbal rubs when I had chest infections or colds as a child, and using steam inhalations to help clear my sinuses, but back then I didn't understand why they worked. Commonly used essential oils for respiratory health include pine (*Pinus sylvestris*), rosemary (*Salvia rosmarinus*) and eucalyptus (*Eucalyptus globulus*) due to their expectorant, antibacterial and antiviral properties. They can also be inhaled and applied as a balm to prevent infection from taking hold. For detailed information on these oils, please refer to the plant profiles in Chapter 6.

Breathe and Release
Chest Rub Recipe

A healing, airway-opening balm to help relieve congestion in the nose and chest, and help support recovery from infection.

YOU WILL NEED

> 5 x sterilised 60ml (2fl oz) tins/jars (not plastic) or one 300ml (10fl oz) jar

> Heat-proof glass jug

> Wooden spoon

> Stirrer/stick (not plastic)

> Heat proof spatula

> Small saucepan

> Water

> Hob

> Food/milk thermometer (optional)

> Essential oils of eucalyptus (*Eucalyptus globulus*), pine (*Pinus sylvestris*), rosemary (*Salvia rosmarinus*)

> 42g (1½oz) beeswax or soy wax pellets (this helps set the balm)

> 252ml (8½fl oz) cold-pressed base (carrier) oil, You can combine base oils to reach a total of 252ml.

Safety Notes

Rosemary essential oil is unsuitable for babies and children as it can restrict their breathing and can be dangerous. Rosemary should also be avoided during pregnancy or while breastfeeding. Those with epilepsy or experiencing fever should not use rosemary oil.

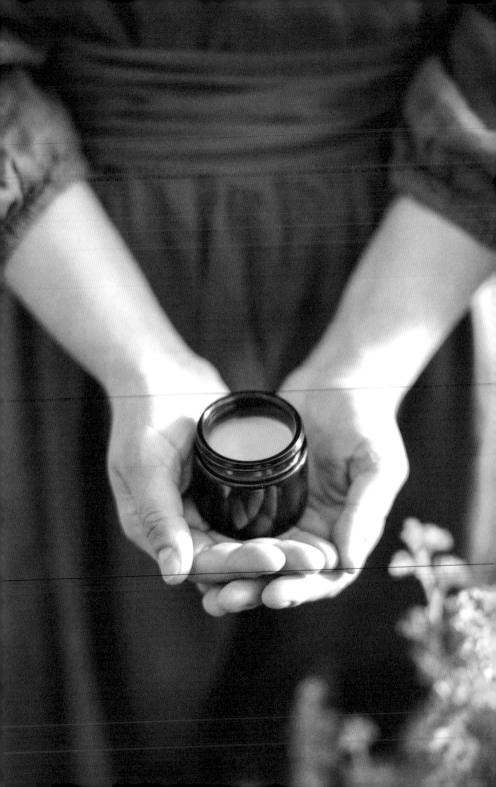

METHOD

1 Bring a saucepan a quarter to a half full of water to a simmer, then reduce the heat to sit just below simmer (85-96°C/185-205°F).

2 Add the base oils to the heat-proof glass jug and place into the pan of water, creating a bain-marie or double-boiler.

3 Heat the base oils gently, stirring occasionally. Make sure no water gets into the jug containing the oils.

4 Add the beeswax pellets to the mixture, stir until melted and combined.

5 Turn off the heat, and using a heat-proof cloth or oven glove, remove the bain-marie from the pan and place onto a heat-proof mat or tea towel to cool.

6 When cooled to approx 57°C (135°F), it is time to add the essential oils to the mix and stir with your stick until well combined (approx 30-60 seconds).

7 Add up to 118 drops of essential oil in total – approximately 6ml (³⁄₁₆fl oz), i.e. a dilution of 2% – consisting of 38 drops of rosemary, 40 of pine, 40 of eucalyptus.

8 Before the mixture cools, pour carefully into your sterilised pots and leave somewhere clean and dry to cool for approx 30 minutes. Don't add it to the fridge – it may cool too quickly and could crystallise, affecting the texture.

9 Once cooled, put on the lids and label your products.

To store, keep in a cool, dark place with the lids tightly on for about six months to a year. To use, apply in circular motions to the affected area up to three times per day, and allow it to penetrate into the skin.

Tip: Warming the affected area with a hot water bottle or a hot flannel first can aid absorption.

CIRCULATORY SYSTEM

Cold weather can exacerbate symptoms of poor peripheral circulation, but the good news is that several essential oils are known for their circulatory stimulant properties. I have made a version of the following recipe for many of my clients who suffer from poor circulation or Raynaud's disease in winter. The essential oils in it bring more blood to the peripheral blood vessels and as such can help to prevent or treat cold, stiff digits, pain, and numbness. This balm can also be used on stiff, tired muscles to warm them and aid recovery post-exercise or after cold exposure.

Keep Warm Balm Recipe

A warming balm to boost peripheral circulation and support muscle recovery.

YOU WILL NEED

> Essential oils of black pepper (*Piper nigrum*), rosemary (*Salvia rosmarinus*), eucalyptus (*Eucalyptus globulus*), marjoram (*Origanum majorana*)

> 5 x sterilised 60ml (2fl oz) tins or glass jars (not plastic). Make sure they are clean; you can sterilise them by putting them in the oven for 10-15 minutes at 160°C (320°F) then soaking the lids in just-boiled water for the same amount of time.

> Heat-proof glass jug

> Wooden spoon

> Stirrer /stick (not plastic)

> Heat-proof spatula

> Small saucepan

> Water

> Hob

> Food/milk thermometer (optional)

> 42g (1½oz) beeswax or soy wax pellets (this helps set the balm)

> 252ml (8½fl oz) cold-pressed base (carrier) oil. You can combine base oils to reach a total of 252ml.

METHOD

1   Bring a saucepan a quarter to a half full of water to a simmer, then reduce the heat to sit just below simmer (85-96°C/185-205°F).

2   Add the base oils to the heat-proof glass jug and place into the pan of water, creating a bain-marie or double-boiler.

3   Heat the base oils gently, stirring occasionally. Make sure no water gets into the jug containing the oils

4   Add the beeswax pellets to the mixture, stir until melted and combined

5   Turn off the heat, and using a heat-proof cloth or oven glove, remove the bain-marie from the pan and place onto a heat-proof mat or tea towel to cool

6   When cooled to approx 57°C (135°F), it is time to add the essential oils to the mix and stir with your stick until well combined (approx 30-60 seconds).

7   Add up to 118 drops of essential oil in total – approximately 6ml (³⁄₁₆fl oz), i.e. a dilution of 2% – consisting of 29 drops of black pepper, 29 drops of rosemary, 30 drops of eucalyptus and 30 drops of marjoram.

8   Before the mixture cools, pour carefully into your sterilised pots and leave somewhere clean and dry to cool for approx 30 minutes. Don't add it to the fridge – it may cool too quickly and could crystallise, affecting the texture.

9   Once cooled, put on the lids and label your products

To store, keep in a cool, dark place with the lids tightly on for about six months to a year. To use, apply in circular motions to the affected area as needed, and allow it to penetrate into the skin.

Tip: warming the affected area with a hot water bottle or hot flannel first can aid absorption, and wearing socks or gloves on top can also help.

Safety Notes

Rosemary essential oil is unsuitable for babies and children as it can dangerously restrict their breathing. It should be avoided during pregnancy or while breastfeeding. Those with epilepsy or experiencing fever should not use rosemary oil. This balm may irritate eyes and delicate skin so only use sparingly on unbroken skin, avoiding the face.

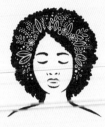

Aromatic Self-care: Support for Mental and Emotional Wellbeing

One of the brilliant things about aromatherapy for emotional wellbeing is that it's very transportable and discreet to use, and therefore easy to call on when we're out and about. I have created three blends below, one is a pulse point roll-on designed to aid with studies or work by lifting the mood whilst improving focus, memory and concentration, another is an 'emotional first aid' inhaler blend which can be called on in times of anxiety, low mood or stress, to soothe the nervous system and help restore calm, and the last one is an energising and uplifting inhaler blend, for when you need a bit of an emotional or energy lift. All the oils in these blends have been chosen and combined especially for their various and complementary actions on the emotional and physical mind. Please see the plant profiles in Chapter 6 for more information on the specific properties of each oil.

Safety Notes

While aromatherapy can be very supportive and help to regulate emotions, it is not a replacement for professional acute mental health support. If you or someone you know is experiencing a mental health crisis please call 999 for emergency support. If you require further mental health support or information, you can find a list of resources in the back of this book.

Never apply essential oils undiluted to skin. Do not use oils that have oxidised (gone off) as this may cause irritation. Usually, this happens with old essential oils that have been exposed to air or heat, and have deteriorated. You can usually smell if an oil has gone bad.

Clarity and Focus Rollerball Recipe

A blend for studying, focusing, remembering or concentrating.

YOU WILL NEED

- 10ml (⅓fl oz) empty glass rollerball bottle

- 10ml (⅓fl oz) base (carrier) oil of your choice. You can use any of the base oils suggested in the carrier oils information section (see Chapter 4)

- Essential oils of rosemary (*Salvia rosmarinus*), pine (*Pinus sylvestris*) and bitter orange (*Citrus × aurantium* var. *Amara*)

- Small measuring jug (25-50ml (1-2fl oz) if possible, or use a small bottle if not available)

- Small funnel to fit the rollerball bottle (if not available, use a small bottle and pour carefully)

- Teaspoon

- Label and pen

METHOD

1 Measure 10ml (⅓fl oz) of your base oil into the small measuring jug.

2 Add up to four drops of each essential oil to the jug, making a total of 12 drops, counting them carefully as you add them.

3 Mix well for 60 seconds with the teaspoon.

4 Remove the lid and ball part of the rollerball bottle.

Safety Notes

Rosemary essential oil is unsuitable for babies and children as it can restrict their breathing and can be dangerous. Rosemary should also be avoided during pregnancy or while breastfeeding. Those with epilepsy or experiencing fever should not use rosemary oil.

5 Using the funnel, decant the mixture into the rollerball bottle.

6 Replace the ball and lid.

7 Label and date your blend.

8 To use, apply to wrists and temples where the skin is thinner and the essential oils will be able to pass through into the bloodstream more easily. You'll also be able to inhale the oils as they absorb into your skin. Make sure you avoid the eyes and other areas of the face.

You can use this blend as needed whenever you need to concentrate on a cognitive task or focus for a long period of time, revise for an exam, or prepare for a job interview, for example. Rosemary has been shown to improve memory[207] and strengthen blood circulation.[208] Pine is invigorating for the mind as well as being an excellent decongestant,[209] and bitter orange is an anxiolytic (has anti-anxiety effects).[210]

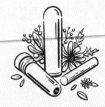

Keep Calm Inhaler Recipe

To help with anxiety and stress, and to soothe the nervous system before a big day or event.

YOU WILL NEED

> Aroma inhaler stick (these can be sourced from online retailers)

> Essential oils of lavender (*Lavandula angustifolia*), lemon balm (*Melissa officinalis*), German chamomile (*Matricaria chamomilla*) and vetiver (*Chrysopogon zizanioides*)

> Tweezers

> A shot glass or small pot

> Label

> Pen

METHOD

1 Take your tweezers and remove the wick from inside the inhaler, placing it into the shot glass or pot.

2 Add three drops of each essential oil to the top of the wick, making a total of 12, counting the drops carefully as you add them.

3 Allow a couple of minutes for the oils to soak down the length of the wick.

4 Use the tweezers to place the wick inside the inhaler stick with the hole, and snap on the round cap at the end.

5 Snap or twist on the lid of the inhaler stick.

6 Label your blend with the names of the essential oils and the date.

7 To use, remove the lid and inhale one to two centimeters from your nose, as needed. Never insert the inhaler into your nose.

Inhalers are a long-lasting and practical way to carry aromatherapy with you. You can take this inhaler with you in a bag or pocket, or keep it in a bedside table. It will last around six months if stored in a cool, dark place with the lid securely on. Once it no longer smells strongly, you can remove the cap and wick, and replace it with a fresh wick and essential oils.

Safety Notes

Lemon balm essential oil (Melissa) should be used at a dilution of 1%
or less for topical (skin) preparations. Lemon balm essential oil
should not be used during pregnancy or if breastfeeding.

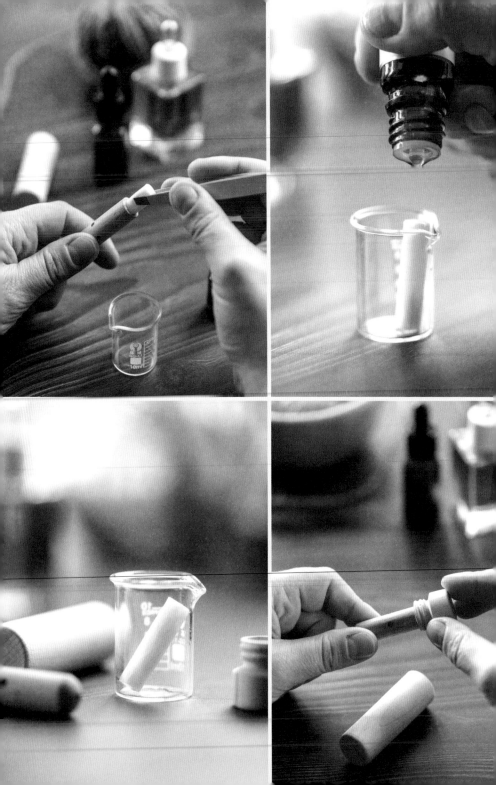

Energising Uplifting Inhaler Recipe

For a little lift when feeling foggy-headed, sluggish or down in the dumps.

YOU WILL NEED

- Essential oils of bergamot (*Citrus × bergamia*), Pine (Pinus sylvestris) and vetiver (*Chrysopogon zizanioides*)
- Inhaler stick and wick
- Labels
- Pens
- Tweezers
- A shot glass or small pot
- Cup of warm/hot water (for warming the vetiver oil)

METHOD

1. Vetiver is a thick, resinous oil and can be tricky to decant, so it is best to pre-warm your bottle of it in a cup of hot water. Make sure the lid is watertight.

2. Using your tweezers, place the inhaler wick into a shot glass, or small pot.

3. Add up to a total of 12 drops of essential oil, from those listed above, to the end of the wick – it will absorb the oils. If you'd like a balanced blend, you could split the oils evenly, adding three drops of each, but if you'd like to include more of the therapeutic properties of a specific oil, you may want to shift the balance slightly.

4. Once the oils have soaked into the wick, pick it up with your tweezers and gently place it inside the inhaler tube (the part with the hole) and snap on the cap.

5. Screw on the lid, and then clearly label your blend with the ingredients, name of the blend (you can be creative here) and the date made.

This blend is energising and uplifting with a grounding element. Your inhaler should last for six months if stored with the lid tightly on, in a cool dark place. Keep it to hand for an uplifting mood boost, and replace the wick with a fresh one when needed.

Safety Notes

Bergamot is photosensitising due to its bergapten content and can therefore irritate the skin. Do not use on skin prior to sun or UV exposure.

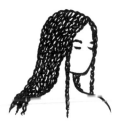

Skincare and Aromatherapy: What Does Smell Have to do With Skin?

While essential oils can have amazing effects on our nerves, breathing, muscles and circulation, they can also help to play an important role in healing and rejuvenating our skin. We've already explored some carrier oils that have skin-healing benefits, but here is a facial oil recipe that contains some essential oils which can be safely used on a regular basis to nourish, soften and reduce inflammation.

Facial Oil Recipe

To soften, rejuvenate and calm, and encourage a healthy glow. This recipe can be adapted for drier or oilier skin types by swapping out the carrier oil for a lighter (for oiler skin) or heavier (for dry skin) option from those in the carrier oils section, or from the two suggested below.

SENSITIVE OR ACNE-PRONE SKIN

Jojoba (*Simmondsia chinensis*) oil can be a good option for psoriasis, eczema or acne-prone skin, since it is technically a wax and is chemically and physically very similar to skin's natural sebum. It is not too 'oily' and may be better tolerated by the skin.

MATURE OR AGEING SKIN

For mature or ageing skin, rosehip seed oil (*Rosa canina*) can be a good choice. Extracted from the seed of the wild dog rose fruit, it is high in essential fatty acids which helps keep cells strong to maintain skin health. It is also rich in antioxidants which can help both prevent and repair skin damage.

YOU WILL NEED

> Essential oils of rose geranium (*Pelargonium graveolens*), lavender (*Lavandula angustifolia*), German chamomile (*Matricaria chamomilla*)

> Carrier oil(s) of your choice

> 30ml (1fl oz) amber glass bottle with dropper (sterilised)

> 50ml (1¾fl oz) measuring beaker or jug

> Small funnel

> Label and pen

METHOD

1 Pour 30ml (1fl oz) total of base oil into the beaker.

2 Add nine drops in total of the three essential oils to the beaker, i.e. three drops each of rose geranium, lavender and German chamomile, and stir to combine.

3 Once combined, use the funnel and pour your mixture into your sterilised bottle.

To use, apply a few drops to your clean fingertips in the morning (or at night, if using rosehip seed oil). Store in a cool, dark place with the lid securely on to prevent oxidation. The oil will last for approximately six months but you'll likely use it up long before then!

Safety Notes

Rosehip seed oil is high in vitamin A (retinol) which encourages skin cell turnover, helping the complexion to look fresh and revitalised, but it can be irritant, so do take care. If you choose this oil, I recommend using 30% rosehip seed oil with a milder carrier oil like sweet almond for the remaining 70% to reduce the chance of irritation. Make sure you do a patch test on the skin before you apply it to your face. Retinol is not safe to use during the daytime as it increases your skin's sensitivity to sunlight, so only use it at night.

The skin of the face is much more delicate than elsewhere on the body so this recipe is a milder 1% blend.

SKINCARE STARTS FROM WITHIN

While many of us apply products galore to our skin day and night, we shouldn't forget that skin health starts from the inside. Here is a recipe for a cold infusion using aromatic herbs that you can drink to support your skincare routine. These herbs have been specially selected for their skin-healing benefits, nutritional content, ability to help clear waste from the body, and/or flavour.

Cold Infusion Recipe for Skin

YOU WILL NEED

> Fridge

> Measuring spoons

> Tea strainer

> Large 1L (34fl oz) jar with lid

> Water

Dried herbs:

> 1 tsp pot marigold, or calendula (*Calendula officinalis*)

> 1 tsp rose petals (*Rosa × damascena*)

> 1 tsp nettle leaves (*Urtica dioica*) – mineral-rich, diuretic[211]

Fresh herbs (where available):

> A few sprigs of peppermint (*Mentha × piperita*), washed and chopped – antiseptic, calming for the digestive system, anti-itch[212]

> A small bunch of cleavers (*Galium aparine*), washed and chopped – diuretic, astringent[213]

> Cucumber slices

> Ice

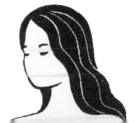

METHOD

1 Measure out all the herbs and add them to your jar.

2 Cover with water and seal the lid.

3 Shake to combine.

4 Place in fridge for 10-12 hours (perhaps overnight).

5 Open the jar and strain into a glass, adding ice cubes and a slice of cucumber if you like.

Safety Notes

Calendula oil is safe for use externally but internal use of the herb should be avoided in pregnancy.

Cleavers are best used fresh and can be foraged but make 100% sure you know the plant and that you're foraging from a safe, legal and clean area. For more guidance see Chapter 7. Peppermint (herb or essential oil) should not be used during pregnancy or if breastfeeding.

Massage and Aromatherapy

Massage is not only enjoyable and relaxing, but reduces tension in the muscles, promotes better circulation and warms the skin, allowing improved absorption of essential oil blends. All of this combined can contribute to healthy, glowing skin. Below, you'll find a QR code to a bonus facial self-massage tutorial which has been designed to do all of these things. Use a few drops of your facial oil and give it a go – a mini-facial that you can do in fifteen minutes.

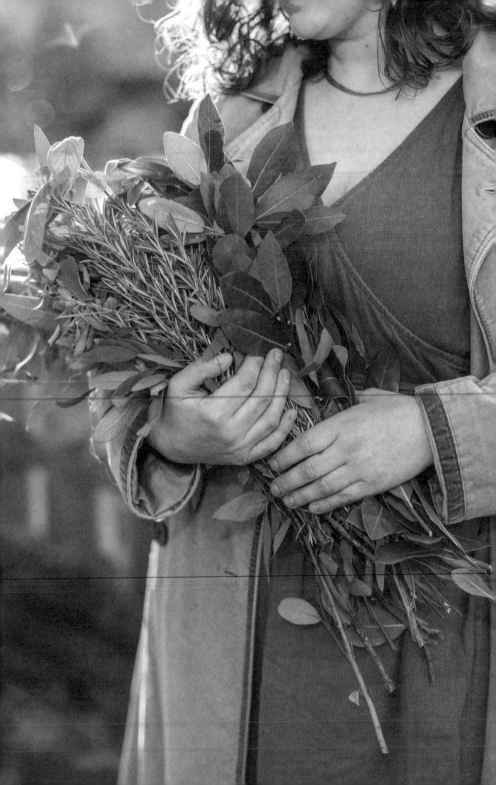

CHAPTER 6
Plant Profiles

"There were strange, rare odors abroad—a tangle of the sea smell and of weeds and damp, new-plowed earth, mingled with the heavy perfume of a field of white blossoms somewhere near." The Awakening, Kate Chopin[214]

In the following pages, you'll find a short overview of 15 of the essential oils that come from the plants I consider some of the most useful when starting out with aromatic explorations. By no means do I suggest that you buy all of them, but the profiles may provide a useful starting point when you wish to choose a couple to begin experimenting with. I have mostly selected some of the more accessibly priced oils that can be grown and sourced from easily accessible locations, although one or two come from further afield or are more pricey, and should be used sparingly and with respect. I have made every effort to make sure that the plants included here are not at risk of becoming endangered, although the situation is always changing, so it's a good idea to consult sources like the IUCN (International Union for Conservation of Nature) red list to make sure that a given plant is not at risk before purchasing essential oils and other ingredients.

Some of the information and guidance on the plant profile pages is collated from a range of reputable sources. These are specified and cited in the resources section at the end of this book for reference.

Bergamot (Citrus × bergamia)

From the citrus family, bergamot oil is zesty, full of sunshine and packs a punch due to its high monoterpene content. Research shows that essential oils, such as bergamot, that contain linalool can act on GABA (gamma-aminobutyric acid – a neurotransmitter) receptors, imparting an anxiolytic (anti-anxiety) and antidepressant effect.

Part used
Rind (peel)

Actions
Calming, uplifting, antispasmodic, and antibacterial

Uses
Anxiety, emotional stress and stress-related digestive issues. Tension, irritability and pent-up stress.

Energetics and symbolism
Traditionally considered a cold and dry oil, but for me, bergamot symbolises gentle warmth and sunshine.

Scent
Fresh, invigorating, slightly floral and citrussy, light

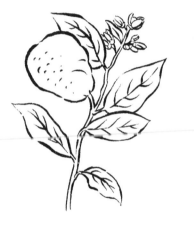

Safety Notes

Bergamot essential oil is phototoxic – do not apply to the skin before exposure to sunlight or UV light. Watch out for oils with a high monoterpene content as they can oxidise easily. If this happens, do not use.

Bitter Orange *(Citrus × aurantium* var. *amara)*

Another citrus oil, this bright, fresh and juicy oil is known for being a 'top note' with its zingy, immediate aroma, which is due to its high monoterpene content. This oil is considered anti-ageing for skin and is especially useful for oily skin types.

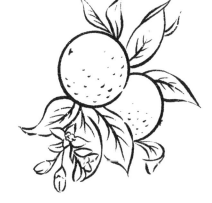

Part used
Rind (peel)

Actions
Astringent, anticoagulant, anti-inflammatory, hypotensive (lowers blood pressure), tonic and regenerative for cells

Uses
Toning the skin, for anxiety, to refresh the spirit, as a circulatory stimulant, and to support metabolism

Energetics and symbolism
To me, orange is the smell of early summer. Energetically it is considered neutral in terms of temperature and moisture, but I find it warming, stimulating and energising.

Scent
Strong, punchy, sharp, warm, opening

Safety Notes
Can cause skin sensitivity as it is phototoxic. Avoid application prior to UV light exposure. Watch out for oils with a high monoterpene content as they can oxidise easily. If this happens, do not use.

Black Pepper *(Piper nigrum)*

An instantly-recognisable oil, black pepper immediately fills the nose with its fizzy, spicy aroma. An invigorating, stimulating oil, it has some very strong actions – go easy with it at first!

Part used
The fruit, or peppercorns

Actions
Anti-inflammatory, analgesic (pain-relieving), antiseptic, cardiac and reproductive stimulant and antispasmodic

Uses
Back pain, stiff muscles, rheumatoid and osteoarthritis, poor circulation, to stimulate digestion, for neuralgia (nerve pain) and to lower fevers. Emotionally, it can be used for a 'boost', to strengthen and fortify the spirits.

Energetics and symbolism
Hot, dry. I see this oil as an immediate energy injection – it doesn't hold back! I use it in my massage clinic for clients who are feeling stiff, sluggish, tired and chilly, particularly in the winter.

Scent
Spicy, strong, heady, fizzy, stimulating, hot, awakening. An upfront, immediate aroma.

Safety Notes

This oil can be irritant so use with caution. Try using it at a low dose of 1% to start with.

Cedar Atlas *(Cedrus atlantica)*

Cedarwood is a gorgeous, rich, resinous oil taken from the distilled wood of the tree. As such it should be used sparingly and with respect since the tree is cut in order to produce the oil. It gives a lovely, grounding and supportive character to blends. Look out for the tree's generous, swooping boughs and bluish-tinged needles.

Part used
Wood

Actions
Anti-inflammatory, balances sebum in skin, decongestant (helps expel mucus from the respiratory system), anti-fungal, reduces tension and stress

Uses
Calming the nerves, for coughs and colds, for feeling grounded, to treat oily skin, and for stimulating lymphatic circulation

Energetics and symbolism
Hot, dry. The majestic stature of the cedar tree invokes stability, confidence, rootedness and strength.

Scent
Reminiscent of forest air, earthy wood, amber, sharp pine and crisp, dry leaves. Fresh, clear aroma with deep, woody undertones.

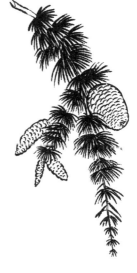

Safety Notes
No known safety issues with topical application of this oil.

Eucalyptus (*Eucalyptus globulus*)

You may have come across this essential oil as an ingredient in various famous chest rubs and balms that are widely sold to relieve coughs and colds. This Australian tree's oil has become a staple in many households across the world for its effectiveness in treating wintertime respiratory illnesses.

Part used
Leaves, twigs

Actions
Antiviral, decongestant, stimulant, anti-inflammatory, antiseptic, antitussive (relieves coughs), insect repellent, lowers fevers

Uses
Coughs and colds, since it opens the airways and expels mucus. Also used for arthritis and fevers. Emotionally it helps to clear the mind and re-invigorate the mood. It is used for those who feel trapped and under pressure, creating space and a sense of openness.

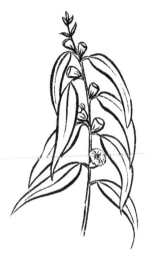

Energetics and symbolism
Warm and dry, this oil has a powerful action on the lungs, both literally and figuratively. It is opening and creates a sense of expansiveness, clearing away negativity.

Scent
Minty, herbaceous, dry, fresh. Spicy, almost lemony. Smells like a hot day, woodchip, and mountain air.

Safety Notes
No known safety issues with topical application of this oil.
Poisonings have been reported due to ingestion.

German Chamomile *(Matricaria chamomilla)*

This oil is like a warm hug and a mug of something hot when I need it most. A flowering plant that grows in dry environments, its friendly yellow-and-white flower is as sweet and soothing as it looks. An excellent oil for calming both the nervous and digestive systems, it has a rich, blue hue due to the chamazulene which forms due to distillation.

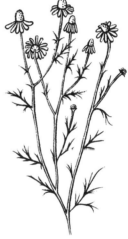

Part used
Flowers

Actions
Strongly anti-inflammatory. Calming for the nerves, digestive tonic, soothing for the skin

Uses
Anxiety, assisting acceptance, stress, fevers, overcoming control issues, digestive irritation, inflammatory skin conditions and allergies including hayfever, asthma and eczema

Energetics and symbolism
Traditionally considered cold and of neutral moisture, to me this herb feels slightly warm and gives a feeling of deep cosiness. I associate this plant with the voice inside (that I often ignore) that is telling me to rest, and accept what I cannot change.

Scent
Sweet, light, warm and apple-y, with a mildly bitter undertone. Smells like freshly-baked biscuits, hay, and honey. Chamomile has the interesting ability to combine a rich biscuity scent with a light, floral, delicate note.

Safety Notes
Generally considered safe for topical application but may irritate some people with allergies to the *Asteraceae* (daisy) family.

Lavender (Lavandula angustifolia)

Probably the most famous of essential oils, and with good reason. Lavender is, I feel, the grandmother of essential oils, and the plant is cultivated all over the world. Curiously, its aroma varies widely depending on the altitude and environment in which it grows.

Part used
Flowering tops

Actions
Strongly anti-inflammatory, analgesic (pain-relieving), and sedative. Antidepressant, anti-inflammatory, antiseptic, antispasmodic.

Uses
Anxiety, insomnia, headaches, infections, minor burns, panic, frustration, IBS, period pains, asthma

Energetics and symbolism
Considered cold and dry. This is one of the best essential oils for 'bringing down heat', whether physically or emotionally. Has a soothing, grandmotherly energy.

Scent
Heady, rich, dry, sweet, floral, minty and herbaceous. Evokes clean washing and gardens.

Safety Notes
No known safety issues with topical application of this oil.

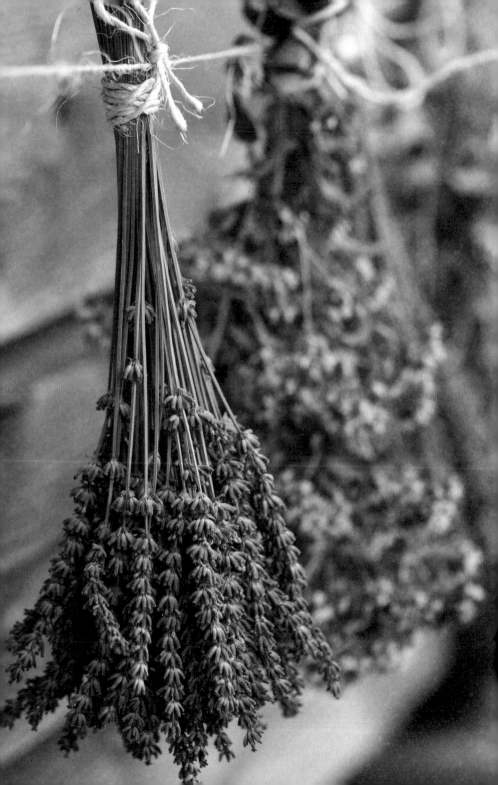

Lemon Balm *(Melissa officinalis)*

Lemon balm is a herb beloved by bees – its Latin name 'Melissa' actually comes from the Greek word for honey bee. It's a cheerful, light herb with a fresh aroma and a ability to lift the spirits. It's a great plant to grow at home, since it supports pollinators and makes a useful kitchen medicine herb, too.

Part used
Flowers and leaves

Actions
Anti-depressive, antiviral, calming, hypotensive (lowers blood pressure), antispasmodic, sedative, lowers fever, anti-inflammatory

Uses
Anxiety and stress, grief, depression, palpitations, panic, treatment of herpes virus. For clarity and reassurance.

Energetics and symbolism
Cold and dry, this oil seems to lend a friendly shoulder and a lightheartedness. It calms and reassures in a gentle yet upbeat way. Its delicate leaves and sweet flowers that attract the bees seem to imbue it with a cheerful, bee-like energy. The bee does not worry as it buzzes from flower to flower – lemon balm invites us to share in this same lightness of being.

Scent
Lemony, fresh, light, herbaceous. Mildly floral and antiseptic.

Safety Notes

Use at a dilution of 1% or less for topical (skin) preparations. Lemon balm essential oil should not be used during pregnancy or if breastfeeding.

Marjoram (Origanum majorana)

Commonly used as a culinary herb, marjoram is both an invigorating yet relaxing herb. Easy to grow and highly fragrant, it makes a welcome addition to gardens and window boxes. It is used frequently in my massage practice for helping to restore tired or injured muscles.

Part used
Flowers and leaves

Actions
Analgesic, antispasmodic, and hypotensive (lowers blood pressure). It is also antimicrobial

Uses
Muscular cramps, aches and spasms, calming the nervous system, and respiratory infections such as bronchitis. Also used for reducing hyperactivity and processing grief.

Energetics and symbolism
Hot, dry. Similarly to black pepper, marjoram is really useful in cases of chilly, tense or stiff muscles and minds in need of a little invigoration, although it is not as harsh or stimulant.

Scent
Herbaceous, soft, warm, earthy. Reminiscent of dry meadow walks and comfort food.

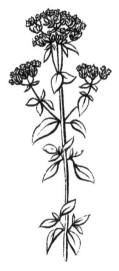

Safety Notes
No known safety issues with topical application of this oil.

Peppermint *(Mentha × piperita)*

Another well-loved and widely-used herb, this is an oil most people will have first smelled in peppermint sweets, cocktails, teas, and toothpaste! However it has uses far beyond the culinary, and will not only freshen the breath but aid the digestion too, and much more besides...

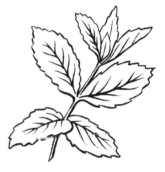

Part used
Flowers and leaves

Actions
Analgesic, antispasmodic, tonic for the nervous system, antifungal, antiseptic, anti-inflammatory, expectorant (expels mucus), supports digestion

Uses
Headaches, coughs, colds, flu and bronchitis, Foggy-headedness, trembling, nervous debility, skin itching or allergies. Used for digestion, both physical and mental (i.e. of ideas, or for processing thoughts and feelings). Peppermint is stimulating and enhances alertness, so is useful in blends for work or study where a clear head is needed.

Energetics and symbolism
Cold, dry. Peppermint is like the cool-headed, clear-thinking friend you need to have around when it's time to make big decisions, focus, and feel alert. It helps process information, soothe headaches and support digestion so that you can get on with what you need to do.

Scent
Fresh, cool, zingy, sharp, refreshing, tingly. Feels like a dip in a cool river, or an ice-cold drink on a hot day.

Safety Notes
Peppermint herb or essential oil should not be used during pregnancy or if breastfeeding.

Pine *(Pinus sylvestris)*

Invigorating, uplifting, and clarifying for the respiratory tract. The 'fresh forest air' feeling that inhaling this oil produces can help to clear the mind and enhance concentration and promote clear-headedness. Several studies suggest that the emotional or physical therapeutic value of Shinrin-yoku (forest bathing, see Chapter 5) lies partially in the inhalation of the essential oils of the trees.

Part used
Needles

Actions
Antibacterial, nervous system tonic, decongestant for the lymphatic system, expectorant (expels mucus), supports adrenal glands, anti inflammatory

Uses
Infections, especially respiratory. To support immunity, boost strength of will and to gently energise. To help expel phlegm from chesty coughs. To uplift and clear the mind without over-stimulating it.

Energetics and symbolism
Hot, dry. To me, the evergreen pine is a symbol of clarity, gentle strength, consistency and continuity. It is both supportive and uplifting.

Scent
Fresh, clarifying, medicinal, invigorating. Like a breath of fresh, forest air.

Safety Notes
No known safety issues with topical application of this oil. Oils with a high monoterpene content can oxidise easily – if this happens, do not use.

Rose (Rosa × damascena)

Known as the queen of flowers, rose has a special place in the hearts of many herbalists and aromatherapists. Almost synonymous with love and the emotional heart, it is probably one of the most powerful yet subtle plants for working with deep-seated emotions. Just being with a rose in the garden can soothe the spirits.

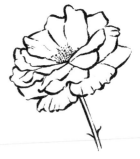

Part used
Flowers (the rosehip fruits and seeds are also used in herbal preparations, but the flower produces the essential oil)

Actions
Anti-depressant, astringent, anti-inflammatory, antioxidant, antimicrobial, relaxant, aphrodisiac, hormone-balancing, anticonvulsant

Uses
For skin inflammation, as a hydrosol (aromatic water) or essential oil. For calming nervous tension, anxiety and depression, as well as for treating insomnia and palpitations. Used also for addressing feelings of being 'not enough'.

Energetics and symbolism
Cold, moist. A holy herb, known in Iranian as 'Gol-E-Mohammadi', rose is a well-known symbol of love and beauty. It is considered to be heart-opening, and can be used to bring compassion and love to emotional trauma and suffering. It is energetically cool and moist and is used to support wellbeing and healing in cases of deep emotional despair or trauma.

Scent
Honeyed, rich, heady, sweet, delicate, complex. Evokes a sense of feeling held and protected.

Safety Notes
No known safety issues with topical application of this oil.

Rose Geranium (Pelargonium graveolens)

An excellent alternative to the more expensive rose, geranium essential oil shares many of the same qualities. It has a fresh, floral note and is both hormone-balancing and adaptogenic. As such, it can play a role in supporting people experiencing nervous tension, adrenal burnout and stress.

Part used
Leaves and flowers

Actions
Calming, hormone-balancing (supports adrenal cortex), reproductive decongestant, antidepressant, astringent, anti-inflammatory, antimicrobial, lymphatic decongestant

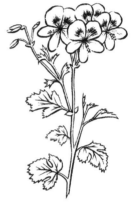

Uses
PMS, burnout, stress, exhaustion and anxiety, especially from being overworked. Also used for treatment of skin conditions like candida, eczema and acne, and to tighten and firm the skin.

Energetics and symbolism
Cold, moist. Native to South Africa, this herb has been a staple in perfumery since the 17th century in Europe, but does not have the long history of medicinal use like some other herbs. For me, therapeutically it symbolises a firm, steadying hand and reassurance in times of emotional turmoil; it has the feeling of a slightly more 'robust rose'. It has a cheerful yet firm disposition.

Scent
Citrussy, heady, strong, bright, rich, dominant

Safety Notes
No known safety issues with topical application of this oil.

Rosemary (Salvia rosmarinus)

This is another well-known culinary herb, native to the Mediterranean area but seen today in gardens all over the world. It has a long history of traditional medicinal and symbolic use as a memory aid, which has been confirmed by modern research. There are many different chemical types of rosemary (called chemotypes) and this variation in chemistry means that care is required when selecting and using the essential oil.

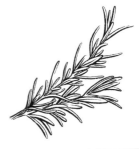

Part used
Leaves

Actions
Central nervous system stimulant, antimicrobial, decongestant, antispasmodic, hypertensive (increases blood pressure), general system tonic

Uses
Relief of stiff, tired muscles, to treat rheumatism, boost circulation in the hands and feet, and boost self-confidence. To support grieving and aid remembrance. As a memory, concentration and study aid.

Energetics and symbolism
Hot, dry. A symbol of remembrance and to support those who are grieving, as well as bringing peace and comfort.

Scent
Powerful, menthol-like, expansive, fortifying, herbaceous, dry. Creates a feeling of focus, determination and strong-willedness.

Safety Notes

Rosemary essential oil is unsuitable for babies and children as it can restrict their breathing and can be dangerous. Rosemary should also be avoided during pregnancy or while breastfeeding. Due to the variation in the different chemotypes, some rosemary oils may be more dangerous in pregnancy, breastfeeding, or for young children, for example the camphor chemotype. Those with epilepsy or experiencing fever should not use rosemary oil.

Vetiver (Chrysopogon zizanioides)

This East Asian oil gives a woody, earthy, and balsamic aroma. Vetiver is a grass, and the essential oil is extracted from the roots of the plant. Known as the 'oil of tranquillity', it induces a feeling of strength, groundedness, stillness, and calm. It is a tonic for the nervous system, and brings a sense of rootedness to blends.

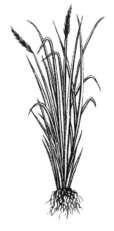

Part used
Roots, sometimes leaves

Actions
Strongly sedative, aphrodisiac, immune tonic, antiseptic, digestive stimulant, hormonal tonic, insect repellent

Uses
Hyperactivity, particularly of the mind, insecurity, severe anxiety, stress, arthritis, rheumatism. Also for inflammatory skin conditions such as acne, dermatitis, and urticaria (itchy, swollen allergic reaction on skin).

Energetics and symbolism
Cold, moist. Traditionally, vetiver root is used to weave insect screens and awnings which emit a gorgeous scent when dampened by the rain. Being a root, this herb's oil brings with it a sense of grounded and rootedness, reconnecting us with the earth when we are caught up in scattered thinking and 'busyness'.

Scent
Earthy, rich, resinous, woody, balsamic. Brings with it a feeling of embodied presence.

Safety Notes
No known safety issues with topical application of this oil.

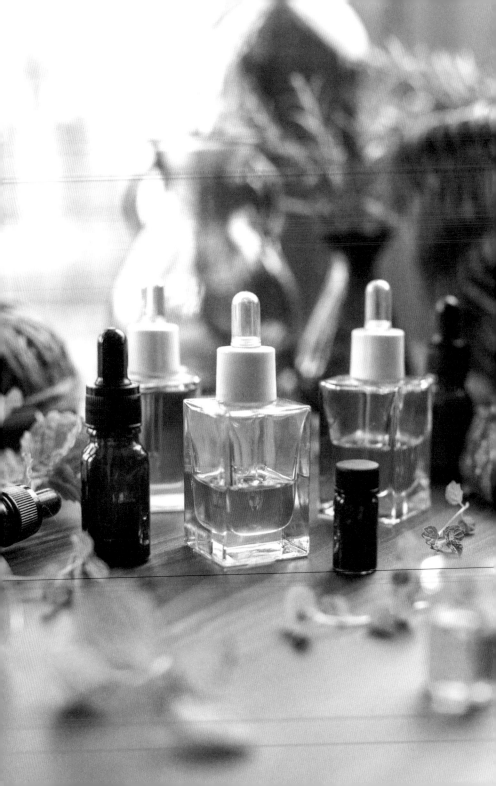

CHAPTER 7
Essential Oil and Herbal Safety

"The persuasive power of an odor cannot be fended off, it enters into us like breath into our lungs, it fills us up, imbues us totally. There is no remedy for it." Perfume: The Story of a Murderer, Patrick Süskind[215]

Throughout this book, you'll see notes about safety alongside recipes and information. These notes are to guide you so that you can use these medicines (because that's what essential oils and herbs are) safely, and with confidence. The information is there not to dissuade you but to aid you as you become more familiar with herbs, essential oils and how to use them.

If you are unsure at any point, you can refer to many of the books, articles and websites that I've included in the Resources and References section at the end of this book to help you. Many of these are sources that I regularly consult in my own practice and I am sure they will be a great support for you as you learn and discover more.

Here is some general guidance which I recommend that you read before you try any recipes or herbal preparations, and refer back to as needed.

DILUTION OF ESSENTIAL OILS

It is really important to dilute essential oils in a base (carrier) oil before use. This is to minimise the risk of allergic reactions. Generally a 1% dilution is advisable for facial products or for those with delicate skin, the elderly or children. For the purposes of massage oil blends, or general-purpose blends for the skin such as body oils or lotions, this is usually a dilution of 2%. This equates to approximately 6 drops of essential oil for 10ml (⅓fl oz) of carrier oil, 12 drops for 20ml (½fl oz), and 18 drops for 30ml (1fl oz). The recipes and activities you'll find in this book all state the percentages and number of drops to use, to guide you if you're new to blending. For guidance on dilution, please refer to a dilution chart such as the one on the Tisserand Institute website (see Resources and References).

INGESTION (EATING OR DRINKING)

Always consult a reputable source to check if a herb is suitable for you before ingesting it (in an infusion, for example). Always consult a qualified medical herbalist if you are not sure about the safety or suitability of a certain herb. Qualified medical herbalists (as opposed to other titles) will have undergone and passed many years of rigorous health, safety, herbal and clinical training. This is important if you do decide to consult a professional for health reasons, as there are many types of herbalists out there with varying levels of knowledge and skill. If you're not sure, NIMH (The National Institute of Medical Herbalists) is a well-regarded professional accreditation body for medical herbalists and has a 'find a herbalist' tool. Similarly, IFPA (the International Federation of Professional Aromatherapists) is an accrediting body for professional aromatherapists and has a tool where you can search for a practitioner in your area.

Essential oils should not be ingested, whether undiluted (neat) or diluted, unless under the guidance of a professional medical aromatherapist or medical herbalist, since they can cause damage to mucous membranes such as the digestive tract. Herbal infusions are your best bet when it comes to ingesting essential oils since you'll derive many of the benefits this way, but please consult a herbalist and do your own research to make sure any herb you consume is safe for you. Never consume macerated oils – this is particularly important if you use fresh plant matter, since a bacteria which causes botulism can grow in the oil and is extremely toxic, even causing death.[216]

PHOTOTOXICITY

This means reactivity to light which can produce undesirable effects. Some base (carrier) oils and essential oils do react with UV light and can cause irritation or more serious effects on the skin so it's important to check before applying. This is another reason why applying neat (undiluted) essential oils to the skin is a bad idea. Any recipes in this book that call for these types of oils have their specific safety information included alongside them to guide you.

IRRITATION

Similarly, essential oils are strong, concentrated plant extracts and as such can produce strong effects. For this reason, always do a patch test on skin with any of the recipes in this book, and discontinue use if irritation occurs. Do not apply essential oils neat (undiluted) to the skin. Some base (carrier) oils may also be irritant for some people. Specific safety information for each oil is included in the carrier oils section (see Chapter 4), so check this before using. Do not use essential or base oils that have oxidised (gone off) as this may cause irritation.

BABIES AND CHILDREN

Caution is needed when using essential oils and herbs with children. Do not use herbs or essential oils with babies or children unless you are under the supervision of a qualified aromatherapist or medical herbalist. It can be dangerous to expose babies and children to certain herbs and oils. Generally speaking, it is wise to avoid using topical (on the skin) essential oil blends of over 1% with children under the age of eight years old, and certain oils should be avoided completely due to the risk of irritation or poisoning. Specific information on the safety of individual essential oils is included throughout the book but if in doubt, please consult a professional aromatherapist or medical herbalist.

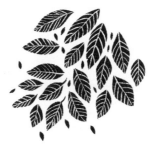

PREGNANCY AND BREASTFEEDING

Caution is also needed when using essential oils and herbs during pregnancy or while breastfeeding. Certain herbs and oils should be avoided completely both for topical and internal use. I have deliberately minimised the inclusion of these herbs and oils in this book, and where these herbs are included, specific safety information is given alongside the recipes.

MEDICATION

The recipes, activities and essential oils included in this book are not a replacement for medical treatment and should not be considered as such. While many oils and herbs have excellent medicinal properties, it is not advisable to make changes to your existing medication or treatment plan unless under the guidance of your doctor, healthcare practitioner and/or a qualified medical herbalist.

SAFE AND ETHICAL PLANT FORAGING

If you are planning to find plants in nature or when out and about, please do your research and make sure you don't pick or smell any toxic or endangered plants or fungi. If you're not 100% sure of a plant's identification, it's best to stick to those you already know for certain are safe, or consult a good identification book. Misidentification can lead to serious poisoning, and some plants look very similar! Alternatively, ask someone trusted who has the right knowledge, or visit a garden where plants are often labelled. Even then, it's best to double-check the identification with someone experienced. Please don't pick plants unless you have to (there's no need to take them home if you are just practising your observation skills for example), and only harvest what you need from a clean, plentiful place for recipes and activities. Thoughtless foraging or picking can disrupt plant growth, damage, or disturb plant population numbers, and uprooting wild plants is against the law in the UK. Please forage mindfully. For more guidance, I'd recommend checking out both the Association of Foragers and the Woodland Trust websites (see Resources and References).

FURTHER READING ON SAFETY

Tisserand and Young have an excellent book on essential oil safety which is included in the resources section of this book, in case you wish to read more on this area. A number of herbal use and safety books are also included.

Resources and References

WEBSITES

AmberLuna Apothecary
www.amberluna.co.uk
This is my website, where you can book workshops and treatments,
or purchase aromatherapy and smell-training kits.

A Modern Herbal
www.botanical.com

Herbal Reality
www.herbalreality.com

IUCN Red List of Threatened Species
iucnredlist.org

Plants of the World Online, Royal Botanic Gardens, Kew
https://powo.science.kew.org/

ARTICLES

Essential oils for restful sleep
herbalreality.com/health-lifestyle/stress-sleep/essential-oils-restful-sleep

Winter warmers: Aromatherapy for respiratory health in cold and flu season
herbalreality.com/herbalism/western-herbal-medicine/winter-warmers-
aromatherapy-for-respiratory-health-cold-flu-season

Essential oils and sustainability: Challenges, opportunities, solutions
herbalreality.com/herbalism/sustainability-social-welfare/essential-
oils-sustainability-challenges-opportunities-solutions

Essential oils for treating inflammation: An aromatherapist's perspective
herbalreality.com/herbalism/western-herbal-medicine/essential-
oils-for-treating-inflammation-aromatherapist-perspective

Healing muscles and joints with essential oils: Recipes from an aromatherapist
herbalreality.com/health-lifestyle/mobility-fitness/
healing-muscles-joints-essential-oils-recipes

BOOKS

Aromatherapy

Worwood, Valerie Ann, *The Fragrant Mind: Aromatherapy for Personality, Mind, Mood, and Emotion*, 2nd edition, Bantam Books, 1997

Mojay, Gabriel, *Aromatherapy for Healing the Spirit: A Guide to Restoring Emotional and Mental Balance through Essential Oils*, Gaia Books, 1999

Herbal medicine

Thomsen, Michael, *The Phytotherapy Desk Reference*, 6th edition, Aeon books, 2022

Bruton-Seal, Julie and Matthew Seal, *Hedgerow Medicine*, Merlin Unwin Books, 2003

Chevallier, Andrew, *Encyclopedia of Herbal Medicine: 550 Herbs and Remedies for Common Ailments*, Dorling Kindersley, 2023

Hoffmann, David, *The Complete Illustrated Holistic Herbal: A Safe and Practical Guide to Making and Using Herbal Remedies*, Element, 1996

Humoural and energetic herbal medicine

Maier, Kat, *Energetic Herbalism: A Guide to Sacred Plant Traditions Integrating Elements of Vitalism, Ayurveda, and Chinese Medicine*, Chelsea Green Publishing, 2022

Hughes, Nathaniel and Fiona Owen *Weeds in the Heart: Explorations in Intuitive Herbalism*, new edition, Aeon Books, 2018

Popham, Sajah, *Evolutionary Herbalism: Science, Spirituality, and Medicine from the Heart of Nature*, North Atlantic Books, 2019

Brooke, Elisabeth, *Traditional Western Herbal Medicine: As above so Below*, Aeon Books, 2019

Plant identification

Rose, Francis and Claire O'Reilly *The Wild Flower Key: How to Identify Wild Plants, Trees and Shrubs in Britain and Ireland*, revised edition, Warne, 2006

Safety

Tisserand, Robert, and Rodney Young, *Essential Oil Safety* 2nd edition, Churchill Livingstone Elsevier, 2014

Scent

Aftel, Mandy, *Essence and Alchemy: A Natural History of Perfume*, Gibbs Smith, 2008

Peace Rhind, Jennifer, *Listening to Scent: An Olfactory Journey with Aromatic Plants and Their Extracts*, Singing Dragon, 2014

McGee, Harold, *Nose Dive: A Field Guide to the World's Smells*, John Murray, 2020

Wellbeing

Hersey, Tricia, *Rest Is Resistance*, The Nap Ministry, 2023

PRACTICAL RESOURCES

The Aromatherapy Trade Council
a-t-c.org.uk

IFPA (International Federation of Professional Aromatherapists)
ifparoma.org

Soil Association
soilassociation.org

Betonica School of Herbal Medicine
betonicaschoolofherbalmedicine.co.uk

NIMH (The National Institute of Medical Herbalists)
nimh.org.uk

Association of Foragers
foragers-association.org

The Woodland Trust
woodlandtrust.org.uk

MENTAL HEALTH

If you or someone you know is experiencing a mental
health crisis or emergency, dial 999.

Mind
mind.org

Mental Health First Aid
MHFAengland.org

Rethink Mental Illness
rethink.org

NHS
nhs.uk/nhs-services/mental-health-services

Samaritans
samaritans.org

Herbs and oils
Baldwins (London) www.baldwins.co.uk
Herbal Apothecary (Yorkshire) www.herbalapothecaryuk.com
Indigo Herbs (Glastonbury) www.indigo-herbs.co.uk
Napiers (Edinburgh) www.napiers.net
Organic Herb Trading (Devon)
Starchild of Glastonbury (Glastonbury) www.organicherbtrading.com
Woodland Herbs (Glasgow) www.woodlandherbs.co.uk

Essential oils and other aromatic ingredients
Amphora Aromatics (Bristol) www.amphora-aromatics.com
Aromantic www.aromantic.co.uk
Materia Aromatica www.materiaaromatica.com
Oshadhi www.oshadhi.co.uk

Thank you to Bristol University Botanical Gardens for allowing us to use their beautiful premises to shoot the photographs in this book.

ESSENTIAL OIL REFERENCES

Below is a list of all sources consulted for the production of the essential oil profile pages. Rather than citing individual sources, I have included a list here, since there is much overlap in the information for each plant.

Battaglia, Salvatore, *Aromatherapy and Shinrin-Yoku* https://salvatorebattaglia.com.au/blog/162-aromatherapy-and-shinrin-yoku

Caddy, Rosemary, *Essential Oils in Colour*, 7th ed, Amberwood Publishing Ltd, Rochester, Kent 1997

Damian, Peter, and Kate Damian, *Aromatherapy: Scent and Psyche*, Healing Arts Press, Rochester, Vermont 1995

Hughes, Nathaniel, *Rose and the Open Door to the Heart*, YouTube, August 13, 2021. https://www.youtube.com/watch?v=oKzKk3tj58s

Mahboubi, Mohaddese, 'Rosa Damascena as Holy Ancient Herb with Novel Applications.' *Journal of Traditional and Complementary Medicine* 6, no. 1 (2016), 10–16. https://doi.org/10.1016/j.jtcme.2015.09.005

Mojay, Gabriel, *Aromatherapy for Healing the Spirit: A Guide to Restoring Emotional and Mental Balance through Essential Oils*, Gaia Books Limited, London 1999

'Relax and Unwind with Forest Bathing', Grow Wild. https://growwild.kew.org/get-involved/resources/how-to/forest-bathing

Rombolà, Laura, Damiana Scuteri, Annagrazia Adornetto, Marilisa Straface, Tsukasa Sakurada, Shinobu Sakurada, Hirokazu Mizoguchi, et al. 'Anxiolytic-like Effects of Bergamot Essential Oil are Insensitive to Flumazenil in Rats.' *Evidence-Based Complementary and Alternative Medicine*, August 14, 2019, 1–6. https://doi.org/10.1155/2019/2156873.

Tisserand, Robert, and Rodney Young, *Essential Oil Safety* 2nd ed, Churchill Livingstone Elsevier, 2014

ENDNOTES

1. 'Scent', *Oxford English Dictionary*, accessed July 20, 2023, https://www.oed.com/search/dictionary/?scope=Entries&q=scent.
2. Matsuo Bashō, *The Narrow Road to the Deep North and Other Travel Sketches* (Harmondsworth, Middlesex: Penguin, 1966), 15.
3. Harold McGee, *Nose Dive: A Field Guide to the World's Smells* (London, UK: John Murray, 2020), xx.
4. Ingrid Martin, *Aromatherapy for Massage Practitioners* (Baltimore, MD: Lippincott Williams & Wilkins, 2007), 27.
5. Charles Spence, 'Musical Scents: On the Surprising Absence of Scented Musical/Auditory Events, Entertainments, and Experiences,' *i-Perception* 12, no. 5 (September 23, 2021), https://doi.org/10.1177/20416695211038747.
6. Ohloff Günther, Wilhelm Pickenhagen, and Philip Kraft, *Scent and Chemistry: The Molecular World of Odors* (Zürich: Verlag Helvetica Chimica Acta, 2012), 24.
7. Helen Keller, *The World I Live In*, version #27683 (London: Hodder & Stoughton, 1908), https://www.gutenberg.org/files/27683/27683-h/27683-h.htm.
8. Aristotle, *Sense and Sensibilia*, trans. J I Beare, 350 BCE, http://classics.mit.edu/Aristotle/sense.2.2.html.
9. Marcel Proust, *Swann's Way (Remembrance of Things Past)*, trans. C K Scott Moncrieff, vol. 1 (Paris: Bernard Grasset, 1913), http://www.authorama.com/remembrance-of-things-past-3.html.
10. Helen Keller, *The World I Live In*, version #27683 (London: Hodder & Stoughton, 1908), https://www.gutenberg.org/files/27683/27683-h/27683-h.htm.
11. Mandy Aftel, *Essence and Alchemy: A Natural History of Perfume* (Layton, UT: Gibbs Smith, 2008).
12. Jonathan Reinarz, *Past Scents: Historical Perspectives on Smell*, Kindle (Chicago, Illinois: University of Illinois Press, 2014), 85-86.
13. Constance Classen, David Howes, and Anthony Synnott, *Aroma: The Cultural History of Smell*, Kindle ed. (London: Routledge, 2002), 3.
14. S. Craig Roberts, Jan Havlíček, and Benoist Schaal, 'Human Olfactory Communication: Current Challenges and Future Prospects,' *Philosophical Transactions of the Royal Society B: Biological Sciences* 375, no. 1800 (2020): p. 20190258, https://doi.org/10.1098/rstb.2019.0258.
15. Constance Classen, David Howes, and Anthony Synnott, *Aroma: The Cultural History of Smell*, Kindle (London: Routledge, 2002), 99.
16. Jonathan Reinarz, *Past Scents: Historical Perspectives on Smell*, Kindle (Chicago, Illinois: University of Illinois Press, 2014), 106.
17. Ibid.
18. Ibid.
19. Avicenna, *Avicenna's Medicine: A New Translation of the 11th-Century Canon with Practical Applications for Integrative Health Care*, trans. M Abu-Asab and M S Micozzi, Kindle Edition (Healing Arts Press, 2013).
20. Helen Keller, *The World I Live In*, version #27683 (London: Hodder & Stoughton, 1908), https://www.gutenberg.org/files/27683/27683-h/27683-h.htm.
21. Harold McGee, *Nose Dive: A Field Guide to the World's Smells* (London, UK: John Murray, 2020), xxi.
22. 'Volatile Definition & Meaning,' Merriam-Webster (Merriam-Webster, 2023), https://www.merriam-webster.com/dictionary/volatile.
23. Jennifer Peace Rhind, *Fragrance and Wellbeing: Plant Aromatics and Their Influence on the Psyche* (London: Singing Dragon, 2014), 19; Christian B. Billesbølle et al., 'Structural Basis of Odorant Recognition by a Human Odorant Receptor,' *Nature* 615 (March 15, 2023): 742–49, https://doi.org/10.1038/s41586-023-05798-y.
24. Amish M. Khan et al., 'Efficacy of Combined Visual-Olfactory Training with Patient-Preferred Scents as Treatment for Patients with COVID-19 Resultant Olfactory Loss,' *JAMA Otolaryngology–Head & Neck Surgery* 149, no. 2 (2023): pp. 141-149, https://doi.org/10.1001/jamaoto.2022.4112.
25. 'Shape Theory of Olfaction,' Shape_theory_of_olfaction (LUMITOS AG, 2023), https://www.chemeurope.com/en/encyclopedia/Shape_theory_of_olfaction.html.
26. John E. Amoore, James W. Johnston, and Martin Rubin, 'The Stereochemical Theory of Odor,' *Scientific American* 210, no. 2 (1964): pp. 42-49, https://doi.org/10.1038/scientificamerican0264-42.
27. Ibid.
28. Jennifer Peace Rhind, *Fragrance and Wellbeing: Plant Aromatics and Their Influence on the Psyche* (London: Singing Dragon, 2014), 20.
29. Ibid.
30. Christian B. Billesbølle et al., 'Structural Basis of Odorant Recognition by a Human Odorant Receptor,' *Nature* 615 (March 15, 2023): 742–49, https://doi.org/10.1038/s41586-023-05798-y.
31. John E. Amoore, James W. Johnston, and Martin Rubin, 'The Stereochemical Theory of Odor,' *Scientific American* 210, no. 2 (1964): pp. 42-49, https://doi.org/10.1038/scientificamerican0264-42.
32. Ingrid Martin, *Aromatherapy for Massage Practitioners* (Baltimore, MD: Lippincott Williams & Wilkins, 2007), 27.
33. V S Ramachandran and Sandra Blakeslee, *Phantoms in the Brain* (New York: William Morrow & Co, 1998), quoted in Ingrid Martin, *Aromatherapy for Massage Practitioners* (Baltimore, MD: Lippincott Williams & Wilkins, 2007), 27.
34. Ingrid Martin, *Aromatherapy for Massage*

Practitioners (Baltimore, MD: Lippincott Williams & Wilkins, 2007), 28.

35. Gordon M Shepherd, 'Perception without a Thalamus,' *Neuron* 46, no. 2 (April 21, 2005): pp. 166-168, https://doi.org/10.1016/j.neuron.2005.03.012.

36. Jennifer Peace Rhind, *Fragrance and Wellbeing: Plant Aromatics and Their Influence on the Psyche* (London: Singing Dragon, 2014), 19.

37. 'Finding Smell Disorders,' AbScent, accessed August 24, 2023, https://abscent.org/. Note that the AbScent charity ceased operations in February 2024.

38. Neisa Santos Pissurno et al., 'Anosmia in the Course of Covid-19,' *Medicine* 99, no. 31 (2020), https://doi.org/10.1097/md.0000000000021280.

39. Ingrid Martin, *Aromatherapy for Massage Practitioners* (Baltimore, MD: Lippincott Williams & Wilkins, 2007), 27.

40. Goran Šimić et al., 'Understanding Emotions: Origins and Roles of the Amygdala,' *Biomolecules* 11, no. 6 (2021): p. 823, https://doi.org/10.3390/biom11060823.

41. Robert M Sargis, 'An Overview of the Pituitary Gland - Endocrineweb,' An Overview of the Pituitary Gland (EndocrineWeb, June 8, 2009), https://www.endocrineweb.com/endocrinology/overview-pituitary-gland.

42. 'Understanding the Stress Response,' *Harvard Health* (Harvard Health Publishing, July 6, 2020), https://www.health.harvard.edu/staying-healthy/understanding-the-stress-response

43. Ibid.

44. Suma P Chand and Raman Marwaha, 'Anxiety,' in *StatPearls* (Treasure Island, FL: StatPearls Publishing, 2022), https://www.ncbi.nlm.nih.gov/books/NBK470361.

45. Bruce S McEwen, 'The End of 'Stress' as We Know It,' The end of 'stress' as we know it | Society for Endocrinology (Society for Endocrinology, 2018), https://www.endocrinology.org/endocrinologist/130-winter18/features/the-end-of-stress-as-we-know-it/.

46. 'Dopamine: What It Is, Function & Symptoms,' Cleveland Clinic, March 23, 2022, https://my.clevelandclinic.org/health/articles/22581-dopamine#:~:text=Dopamine%20is%20also%20a%20neurohormone%20released%20by%20the%20hypothalamus%20in%20your%20brain.

47. Stephanie Watson, 'Dopamine: The Pathway to Pleasure,' Harvard Health (Harvard Health Publishing, July 20, 2021), https://www.health.harvard.edu/mind-and-mood/dopamine-the-pathway-to-pleasure.

48. Stephanie Watson, 'Oxytocin: The Love Hormone,' Harvard Health (Harvard Health Publishing, July 20, 2021), https://www.health.harvard.edu/mind-and-mood/oxytocin-the-love-hormone.

49. Zainab Shahid, Edinen Asuka, and Gurdeep Singh, 'Physiology, Hypothalamus,' accessed February 20, 2023, https://www.ncbi.nlm.nih.gov/books/NBK535380/.

50. Ingrid Martin, *Aromatherapy for Massage Practitioners* (Baltimore, MD: Lippincott Williams & Wilkins, 2007), 28.

51. Asya Rolls, Jana Schaich Borg, and Luis de Lecea, 'Sleep and Metabolism: Role of Hypothalamic Neuronal Circuitry,' *Best Practice & Research Clinical Endocrinology & Metabolism* 24, no. 5 (October 2010): pp. 817-828, https://doi.org/10.1016/j.beem.2010.08.002.

52. Dalinda Isabel Sánchez-Vidaña et al., 'The Effectiveness of Aromatherapy for Depressive Symptoms: A Systematic Review,' *Evidence-Based Complementary and Alternative Medicine* 2017 (January 4, 2017): pp. 1-21, https://doi.org/10.1155/2017/5869315.

53. Michiaki Okuda et al., 'Aromatherapy Improves Cognitive Dysfunction in Senescence-Accelerated Mouse Prone 8 by Reducing the Level of Amyloid Beta and Tau Phosphorylation,' *PLOS ONE* 15, no. 10 (2020), https://doi.org/10.1371/journal.pone.0240378.

54. Yuanguang Ma, 'The Influence of Ambient Aroma on Middle School Students' Academic Emotions,' *International Journal of Psychology* 57, no. 3 (2022): pp. 387-392, https://doi.org/10.1002/ijop.12827.

55. J Lehrner et al., 'Ambient Odor of Orange in a Dental Office Reduces Anxiety and Improves Mood in Female Patients,' *Physiology & Behavior* 71, no. 1-2 (October 2000): pp. 83-86, https://doi.org/10.1016/s0031-9384(00)00308-5.

56. Kenji Yamada et al., 'Effect of Inhalation of Chamomile Oil Vapour on Plasma ACTH Level in Ovariectomized-Rat under Restriction Stress.,' *Biological and Pharmaceutical Bulletin* 19, no. 9 (September 1996): pp. 1244-1246, https://doi.org/10.1248/bpb.19.1244.

57. Mahbubeh Tabatabaeichehr and Hamed Mortazavi, 'The Effectiveness of Aromatherapy in the Management of Labor Pain and Anxiety: A Systematic Review,' *Ethiopian Journal of Health Sciences* 30, no. 3 (May 2020), https://doi.org/10.4314/ejhs.v30i3.16.

58. Ibid.

59. Ingrid Martin, *Aromatherapy for Massage Practitioners* (Baltimore, MD: Lippincott Williams & Wilkins, 2007), 160.

60. Mahbubeh Tabatabaeichehr and Hamed Mortazavi, 'The Effectiveness of Aromatherapy in the Management of Labor Pain and Anxiety: A Systematic Review,' *Ethiopian Journal of Health Sciences* 30, no. 3 (May 2020), https://doi.org/10.4314/ejhs.v30i3.16.

61. Diane Ackerman, *A Natural History of the Senses* (Phoenix, 1996), xvi.

62. Daphne Du Maurier, *Rebecca* (Harmondsworth: Penguin Books Ltd, 1938), https://archive.org/details/in.ernet.dli.2015.461023.

63. 'Limbic System: Structure and Function | Emotion (Video),' Khan Academy (Khan Academy, 2023), https://www.khanacademy.org/test-prep/mcat/processing-the-environment/emotion/v/emotions-limbic-system.

64. Colleen Walsh, 'How Scent, Emotion, and Memory Are Intertwined - and Exploited,' Harvard Gazette (Harvard Gazette, February 27, 2020), https://news.harvard.edu/gazette/story/2020/02/how-scent-emotion-and-memory-are-intertwined-and-exploited/.

65. Afif J. Aqrabawi and Jun Chul Kim, 'Olfactory Memory Representations Are Stored in the Anterior Olfactory Nucleus,' Nature Communications 11, no. 1 (June 2020), https://doi.org/10.1038/s41467-020-15032-2.

66. Ingrid Martin, Aromatherapy for Massage Practitioners (Baltimore, MD: Lippincott Williams & Wilkins, 2007), 29.

67. Bryan Kolb and Robbin Gibb, 'Brain Plasticity and Behaviour in the Developing Brain,' ed. Margaret Clarke and Laura Ghali, Journal of the Canadian Academy of Child and Adolescent Psychiatry (Journal De L'Académie Canadienne De Psychiatrie De L'enfant Et De L'adolescent) 20, no. 4 (November 2011): pp. 265-276, https://doi.org/10.1016/b978-0-444-63327-9.00005-9.

68. A M Mouly and R Sullivan, '15 - Memory and Plasticity in the Olfactory System: From Infancy to Adulthood.,' in The Neurobiology of Olfaction, ed. A Menini (Boca Raton, FL: CRC Press/Taylor & Francis, 2010).

69. Ibid.

70. Ingrid Martin, Aromatherapy for Massage Practitioners (Baltimore, MD: Lippincott Williams & Wilkins, 2007), 29.

71. Ibid.

72. Sam Gochman, 'Scentimental Associations with Nature: Odor-Associative Learning and Biophilic Design,' Terrapin Bright Green (Terrapin Bright Green, May 9, 2016), https://www.terrapinbrightgreen.com/blog/2016/05/scentimental-associations-with-nature/.

73. Mandy Aftel, Fragrant: The Secret Life of Scent (New York, New York: Riverhead Books, 2014), 3.

74. Harold McGee, Nose Dive: A Field Guide to the World's Smells (London, UK: John Murray, 2020), 86.

75. Kurt Schnaubelt, Medical Aromatherapy: Healing with essential oils (Berkley: Frog, 1999).

76. Avicenna, Avicenna's Medicine: A New Translation of the 11th-Century Canon with Practical Applications for Integrative Health Care, trans. M Abu-Asab and M S Micozzi, Kindle Edition (Healing Arts Press, 2013).

77. Yogini S. Jaiswal and Leonard L. Williams, 'A Glimpse of Ayurveda – the Forgotten History and Principles of Indian Traditional Medicine,' Journal of Traditional and Complementary Medicine 7, no. 1 (February 28, 2016): 50–53, https://

78. 'Chinese Medicine,' Johns Hopkins Medicine, December 2, 2019, https://www.hopkinsmedicine.org/health/wellness-and-prevention/chinese-medicine.

79. Elisabeth Brooke, Traditional Western Herbal Medicine: As above so Below (Aeon, 2019).

80. Anwarul Hassan Gilani and Atta-ur Rahman, 'Trends in Ethnopharmacology,' Journal of Ethnopharmacology 100, no. 1–2 (August 22, 2005): 43–49, https://doi.org/10.1016/j.jep.2005.06.001.

81. Ibid

82. Ahmed M. Metwaly et al., 'Traditional Ancient Egyptian Medicine: A Review,' Saudi Journal of Biological Sciences 28, no. 10 (June 19, 2021): 5823–32, https://doi.org/10.1016/j.sjbs.2021.06.044.

83. Mandy Aftel, Fragrant: The Secret Life of Scent (New York, New York: Riverhead Books, 2014), 3.

84. Elise Vernon Pearlstine, Scent: A Natural History of Fragrance (Yale University Press, 2022), 16.

85. Maud Grieve, 'Meadowsweet,' A Modern Herbal, 1995, https://www.botanical.com/botanical/mgmh/m/meadow28.html.

86. Ahmed Essa and Alī Othmān, 'Studies in Islamic Civilization: The Muslim Contribution to the Renaissance,' in Studies in Islamic C0-77, Civilization: The Muslim Contribution to the Renaissance (Herndon, VA: The International Institute of Islamic Thought (IIIT), 2010), 7, https://iiit.org/wp-content/uploads/2018/07/books-in-brief-studies_in_islamic_civilizations.pdf.

87. Gabriel Mojay, Aromatherapy for Healing the Spirit: A Guide to Restoring Emotional and Mental Balance through Essential Oils (London: Gaia Books Limited, 1999), 9.

88. John O'Connell, The Book of Spice: From Anize to Zedoary (London: Profile books, 2016).

89. https://www.worldhistory.org/article/1777/the-spice-trade--the-age-of-exploration/

90. 'Trade History of the Silk Road, Spice & Incense Routes,' Trade History of the Silk Road, Spice & Incense Routes, accessed July 6, 2023, http://www.silkroutes.net/SilkSpiceIncenseRoutes.htm.

91. Elise Vernon Pearlstine, Scent: A Natural History of Fragrance (Yale University Press, 2022), 21.

92. Jennifer Peace Rhind, Listening to Scent: An Olfactory Journey with Aromatic Plants and Their Extracts (London: Singing Dragon, 2014), 41-43.

93. Sajah Popham, Evolutionary Herbalism: Science, Medicine, and Spirituality from the Heart of Nature (Berkeley, CA: North Atlantic Books, 2019), 273-274.

94. Aristotle, Sense and Sensibilia, translated by J I Beare, On Sense and the Sensible by Aristotle, 350AD. http://classics.mit.edu/Aristotle/sense.2.2.html.

95. Sajah Popham, Evolutionary Herbalism: Science, Medicine, and Spirituality from the Heart of Nature (Berkeley, CA: North Atlantic Books, 2019), 322.

96. Juan Favela-Hernández et al., 'Chemistry

and Pharmacology of Citrus Sinensis,' *Molecules* 21, no. 2 (2016): p. 247, https://doi.org/10.3390/molecules21020247.

97. Rosemary Caddy, *Essential Oils in Colour*, 7th ed. (Rochester, Kent: Amberwood Publishing Ltd., 1997), 61.

98. Ingrid Martin, *Aromatherapy for Massage Practitioners* (Baltimore, MD: Lippincott Williams & Wilkins, 2007), 35.

99. Harold McGee, *Nose Dive: A Field Guide to the World's Smells* (London, UK: John Murray, 2020), 169.

100. Ingrid Martin, *Aromatherapy for Massage Practitioners* (Baltimore, MD: Lippincott Williams & Wilkins, 2007), 36.

101. Ibid.

102. Perry Fung Lim, Xiang Yang Liu, and Sui Yung Chan, 'A Review on Terpenes as Skin Penetration Enhancers in Transdermal Drug Delivery,' *Journal of Essential Oil Research* 21, no. 5 (December 8, 2011): pp. 423-428, https://doi.org/10.1080/10412905.2009.9700208.

103. Eng Soon Teoh, 'Secondary Metabolites of Plants,' *Medicinal Orchids of Asia*, November 5, 2015, pp. 59-73, https://doi.org/10.1007/978-3-319-24274-3_5.

104. Arryn Craney, Salman Ahmed, and Justin Nodwell, 'Towards a New Science of Secondary Metabolism,' *The Journal of Antibiotics* 66, no. 7 (2013): Valerie Ann Worwood, *The Fragrant Mind: Aromatherapy for Personality, Mind, Mood, and Emotion*, 2nd ed. (Reading, Berkshire: Bantam books, 1997), 348.

105. Javad Sharifi-Rad et al., 'Biological Activities of Essential Oils: From Plant Chemoecology to Traditional Healing Systems,' *Molecules* 22, no. 1 (January 2017): p. 70, https://doi.org/10.3390/molecules22010070.

106. Abdul Rouf Wani et al., 'An Updated and Comprehensive Review of the Antiviral Potential of Essential Oils and Their Chemical Constituents with Special Focus on Their Mechanism of Action against Various Influenza and Coronaviruses,' *Microbial Pathogenesis* 152 (October 16, 2020): pp. 387-400, https://doi.org/10.1016/j.micpath.2020.104620.

107. Gabriel Mojay, *Aromatherapy for Healing the Spirit: A Guide to Restoring Emotional and Mental Balance through Essential Oils* (London: Gaia Books Limited, 1999), 10.

108. Valerie Ann Worwood, *The Fragrant Mind: Aromatherapy for Personality, Mind, Mood, and Emotion*, 2nd ed. (Reading, Berkshire: Bantam books, 1997), 348.

109. Ingrid Martin, *Aromatherapy for Massage Practitioners* (Baltimore, MD: Lippincott Williams & Wilkins, 2007), 37.

110. Elise Vernon Pearlstine, *Scent: A Natural History of Fragrance* (Yale University Press, 2022), 155.

111. Valerie Ann Worwood, *The Fragrant Mind: Aromatherapy for Personality, Mind,* Mood, and Emotion, 2nd ed. (Reading, Berkshire: Bantam books, 1997), 17.

112. Gabriel Mojay, *Aromatherapy for Healing the Spirit: A Guide to Restoring Emotional and Mental Balance through Essential Oils* (London: Gaia Books Limited, 1999), 10.

113. Rosemary Caddy, *Essential Oils in Colour*, 7th ed. (Rochester, Kent: Amberwood Publishing Ltd., 1997), 1.1.

114. Jugreet Sharmeen et al., 'Essential Oils as Natural Sources of Fragrance Compounds for Cosmetics and Cosmeceuticals,' *Molecules* 26, no. 3 (January 27, 2021): p. 666, https://doi.org/10.3390/molecules26030666.

115. Javad Sharifi-Rad et al., 'Biological Activities of Essential Oils: From Plant Chemoecology to Traditional Healing Systems,' *Molecules* 22, no. 1 (January 2017): p. 70, https://doi.org/10.3390/molecules22010070.

116. Gabriel Mojay, *Aromatherapy for Healing the Spirit: A Guide to Restoring Emotional and Mental Balance through Essential Oils* (London: Gaia Books Limited, 1999), 10.

117. Ingrid Martin, *Aromatherapy for Massage Practitioners* (Baltimore, MD: Lippincott Williams & Wilkins, 2007), 11.

118. Ahmed Essa and Alī Othmān, 'Studies in Islamic Civilization: The Muslim Contribution to the Renaissance,' in *Studies in Islamic Civilization: The Muslim Contribution to the Renaissance* (Herndon, VA: The International Institute of Islamic Thought (IIIT), 2010), pp. 70-77, https://iiit.org/wp-content/uploads/2018/07/books-in-brief_studies_in_islamic_civilizations.pdf.

119. Mohaddese Mahboubi, 'Rosa Damascena as Holy Ancient Herb with Novel Applications,' *Journal of Traditional and Complementary Medicine* 6, no. 1 (2016): pp. 10-16, https://doi.org/10.1016/j.jtcme.2015.09.005.

120. Š Schlosser, 'Distillation – from Bronze Age till Today,' in *Proceedings of the 38th International Conference of Slovak Society of Chemical Engineering* (Bratislava, Slovakia: Institute of Chemical and Environmental Engineering, Slovak University of Technology., 2011), pp. 11-12, https://www.researchgate.net/publication/260392019_Distillation_-_from_Bronze_Age_till_today.

121. Eleanor Beardsley, 'In France's Perfume Capital of the World, There's a World of Beautiful Fragrance,' *NPR* (NPR, September 25, 2021), https://www.npr.org/2021/09/25/1039336681/grasse-perfume-france.

122. Paolo Pallado et al., 'Gas Chromatography/Mass Spectrometry in Aroma Chemistry: A Comparison of Essential Oils and Flavours Extracted by Classical and Supercritical Techniques,' *Rapid Communications in Mass Spectrometry* 11, no. 12 (December 4, 1998): pp. 1335-1341, https://doi.org/10.1002/(sici)1097-0231(199708)11:12<1335::aid-rcm970>3.0.co;2-r.

123. Ingrid Martin, *Aromatherapy for Massage Practitioners* (Baltimore, MD: Lippincott Williams & Wilkins, 2007), 12.

124. Ibid, 13.

125. Preetha Bhadra and Sagarika Parida, eds., *Aromatherapy and Its Benefits*, 1st ed. (New Delhi: Renu Publishers, 2021), https://www.researchgate.net/publication/350038518_Aromatherapy.

126. Wendy Robbins, 'CO2 Supercritical Extract Guide,' AromaWeb, accessed March 31, 2023, https://www.aromaweb.com/articles/whatco2s.asp.

127. Paolo Pallado et al., 'Gas Chromatography/Mass Spectrometry in Aroma Chemistry: A Comparison of Essential Oils and Flavours Extracted by Classical and Supercritical Techniques,' *Rapid Communications in Mass Spectrometry* 11, no. 12 (December 4, 1998): pp. 1335-1341, https://doi.org/10.1002/(sici)1097-0231(199708)11:12<1335::aid-rcm970>3.0.co;2-r.

128. Wendy Robbins, 'What Are Absolutes?,' AromaWeb (AromaWeb), accessed March 31, 2023, https://www.aromaweb.com/articles/whatabso.asp.

129. Erica Bauermeister, *The Scent Keeper* (MacMillan Audio, 2019).

130. Miguel Trancozo Trevino, 'The People Trying to Save Scents from Extinction,' *BBC Future* (BBC, January 13, 2020), https://www.bbc.com/future/article/20200109-why-preserving-certain-scents-is-important.

131. Elise Vernon Pearlstine, *Scent: A Natural History of Fragrance* (Yale University Press, 2022), 155.

132. Ingrid Martin, *Aromatherapy for Massage Practitioners* (Baltimore, MD: Lippincott Williams & Wilkins, 2007), 14.

133. Encyclopædia Britannica, 'Perfume,' *Encyclopædia Britannica* (Encyclopædia Britannica, inc., January 24, 2023), https://www.britannica.com/art/perfume#ref13686.

134. Gabriel Mojay, *Aromatherapy for Healing the Spirit: A Guide to Restoring Emotional and Mental Balance through Essential Oils* (London: Gaia Books Limited, 1999), 12.

135. Ingrid Martin, *Aromatherapy for Massage Practitioners* (Baltimore, MD: Lippincott Williams & Wilkins, 2007), 14.

136. Elise Vernon Pearlstine, *Scent: A Natural History of Fragrance* (Yale University Press, 2022), 155.

137. Kim Walker and Vicky Chown, 'Herbal Infused Oils: Part 1,' Handmade Apothecary (Handmade Apothecary), accessed April 3, 2023, https://www.handmadeapothecary.co.uk/infused-oils-intro.

138. Penny Price, 'Making Macerated Oils,' Penny Price Aromatherapy (Penny Price Aromatherapy, May 10, 2020), https://www.penny-price.com/blogs/news/making-macerated-oils.

139. St. Gelais, Alexis. 'The Highs and Lows of GC-MS in Essential Oil Analysis.' Tisserand Institute, July 15, 2020. https://tisserandinstitute.org/highs-lows-gc-ms-essential-oil-analysis/.

140. Ellen Rowland, 'Essential Oils and Sustainability: Challenges, Opportunities, Solutions,' Herbal Reality, May 10, 2022, https://www.herbalreality.com/herbalism/sustainability-social-welfare/essential-oils-sustainability-challenges-opportunities-solutions/.

141. Gabriel Mojay, *Aromatherapy for Healing the Spirit: A Guide to Restoring Emotional and Mental Balance through Essential Oils* (London: Gaia Books Limited, 1999), 17.

142. 'Ethanol: Paula's Choice,' Paula's Choice Skincare, accessed April 24, 2023, https://www.paulaschoice.com/ingredient-dictionary/ingredient-ethanol.html.

143. Ingrid Martin, *Aromatherapy for Massage Practitioners* (Baltimore, MD: Lippincott Williams & Wilkins, 2007), 29.

144. Vicky Chown and Kim Walker, *The Handmade Apothecary: Healing Herbal Remedies* (London: Kyle Books, 2017), 24.

145. Timothy Miller, 'Skin Deep: Dermal Absorption of Essential Oils,' Naturopathic CE, May 12, 2021, https://www.naturopathicce.com/natnotes/skin-deep-dermal-absorption-of-essential-oils/.

146. Ibid.

147. Ingrid Martin, *Aromatherapy for Massage Practitioners* (Baltimore, MD: Lippincott Williams & Wilkins, 2007), 30.

148. Timothy Miller, 'Skin Deep: Dermal Absorption of Essential Oils,' Naturopathic CE, May 12, 2021, https://www.naturopathicce.com/natnotes/skin-deep-dermal-absorption-of-essential-oils/.

149. Ingrid Martin, *Aromatherapy for Massage Practitioners* (Baltimore, MD: Lippincott Williams & Wilkins, 2007), 30.

150. Annie Hall et al., eds., *Botanical Skin Care Recipe Book* (Bedford, MA: Herbal Academy, 2019), 5.

151. 'Carrier Oils,' Naissance UK, accessed April 24, 2023, https://naissance.com/blogs/naissance-blog/carrier-oils.

152. Diane Ackerman, *A Natural History of the Senses* (London, Phoenix, 1996).

153. Sajah Popham, *Evolutionary Herbalism: Science, Medicine, and Spirituality from the Heart of Nature* (Berkeley, CA: North Atlantic Books, 2019), 286-288.

154. 'Essential Oil Dilution Chart,' Tisserand Institute, December 11, 2020, https://tisserandinstitute.org/essential-oil-dilution-chart/.

155. 'Carrier Oils,' Naissance UK, accessed August 17, 2023, https://naissance.com/blogs/naissance-blog/carrier-oils.

156. 'Avocado Oil: Paula's Choice,' Paula's Choice, accessed August 17, 2023, https://www.paulaschoice.com/ingredient-dictionary/ingredient-avocado-oil.html.

157. Shirley Price and Len Price, *Aromatherapy for Health Professionals*, 4th ed. (Elsevier, 2012), 192.

158. 'Olive Oil/Olive Fruit Oil in Skin Care: What It Is: Paula's Choice,' Paula's Choice, accessed August 17, 2023, https://www.paulaschoice.com/ingredient-

159. 'Olive Oil/Olive Fruit Oil in Skin Care: What It Is: Paula's Choice,' Paula's Choice, accessed August 24, 2023, https://www.paulaschoice.com/ingredient-dictionary/ingredient-olive-oil-olive-fruit-oil.html.

160. Simon G Danby et al., 'Effect of Olive and Sunflower Seed Oil on the Adult Skin Barrier: Implications for Neonatal Skin Care,' Pediatric Dermatology 30, no. 1 (2012): 42–50, https://doi.org/10.1111/j.1525-1470.2012.01063.x.

161. 'Sweet Almond Oil,' Paula's Choice, accessed August 17, 2023, https://www.paulaschoice.co.uk/sweet-almond-oil/ingredient-sweet-almond-oil.html.

162. Shirley Price and Len Price, Aromatherapy for Health Professionals, 4th ed. (Elsevier, 2012), 192.

163. 'Coconut Oil,' Paula's Choice, accessed August 17, 2023, https://www.paulaschoice.com/ingredient-dictionary/ingredient-coconut-oil.html.

164. 'Carrier Oils,' Naissance UK, accessed April 24, 2023, https://naissance.com/blogs/naissance-blog/carrier-oils.

165. Christina L. Burnett et al., 'Final Report on the Safety Assessment of Cocos Nucifera (Coconut) Oil and Related Ingredients,' International Journal of Toxicology 30, no. 3_suppl (2011), https://doi.org/10.1177/1091581811400636.

166. 'Coconut Oil,' Paula's Choice, accessed August 17, 2023, https://www.paulaschoice.com/ingredient-dictionary/ingredient-coconut-oil.html.

167. 'Sunflower Seed Oil,' Paula's Choice, accessed August 17, 2023, https://www.paulaschoice.com/ingredient-dictionary/ingredient-sunflower-seed-oil.html.

168. Shirley Price and Len Price, Aromatherapy for Health Professionals, 4th ed. (Elsevier, 2012), 193.

169. Carole Fisher, Materia Medica of Western Herbs (London, Greater London: Aeon, 2018).

170. Disha Arora, Anita Rani, and Anupam Sharma, 'A Review on Phytochemistry and Ethnopharmacological Aspects of Genus Calendula,' Pharmacognosy Reviews 7, no. 14 (2013): 179, https://doi.org/10.4103/0973-7847.120520.

171. Carole Fisher, Materia Medica of Western Herbs (London, Aeon, 2018).

172. Michael Thomsen, The Phytotherapy Desk Reference, 6th ed. (Aeon Books, 2022), 36.

173. Matsuo Bashō, The Narrow Road to the Deep North and Other Travel Sketches (Harmondsworth, Middlesex, Penguin, 1966), 79.

174. 'Observation', Oxford English Dictionary, accessed December 16, 2023, https://www.oed.com/search/dictionary/?scope=Entries&q=observation dictionary/?scope=Entries&q=observation

175. Peter A. Coventry et al., 'Nature-Based Outdoor Activities for Mental and Physical Health: Systematic Review and Meta-Analysis,' SSM - Population Health 16 (October 1, 2021): 100934, https://doi.org/10.1016/j.ssmph.2021.100934.

176. 'Social Prescribing: The Power of Nature as Treatment,' Natural England, April 12, 2022, https://naturalengland.blog.gov.uk/2022/04/12/social-prescribing-the-power-of-nature-as-treatment/.

177. Salvatore Battaglia, 'Aromatherapy and Shinrin-Yoku,' Salvatore Battaglia, accessed July 25, 2023, https://salvatorebattaglia.com.au/blog/162-aromatherapy-and-shinrin-yoku.

178. Leanne Martin et al., 'Nature Contact, Nature Connectedness and Associations with Health, Wellbeing and pro-Environmental Behaviours,' Journal of Environmental Psychology 68 (January 18, 2020): 101389, https://doi.org/10.1016/j.jenvp.2020.101389.

179. 'Education Is Key to Addressing Climate Change,' United Nations, accessed July 25, 2023, https://www.un.org/en/climatechange/climate-solutions/education-key-addressing-climate-change.

180. 'Olfaction', Oxford English Dictionary, accessed July 20, 2023, https://www.oed.com/search/dictionary/?scope=Entries&q=olfaction.

181. Jennifer Peace Rhind, Fragrance and Wellbeing: Plant Aromatics and Their Influence on the Psyche (London: Singing Dragon, 2014), 44.

182. Isha Tickoo, 'Nature Journaling,' Grow Wild (Royal Botanic Gardens, Kew, December 20, 2021), https://growwild.kew.org/blog/nature-journaling.

183. 'Other Monographs and Articles,' Other monographs and Articles - American Botanical Council, accessed April 26, 2023, https://www.herbalgram.org/resources/other-monographs-and-articles/.

184. 'A Curious Herbal - Dandelion,' British Library, accessed April 26, 2023, https://www.bl.uk/collection-items/a-curious-herbal-dandelion.

185. Maude Grieve, A Modern Herbal, 1931, https://botanical.com/.

186. Jennifer Peace Rhind, Fragrance and Wellbeing: Plant Aromatics and Their Influence on the Psyche (London: Singing Dragon, 2014), 146.

187. 'Principles of Practice,' The Association of Foragers - Principles, March 18, 2019, https://foragers-association.org/principles.

188. 'Foraging Guidelines,' Woodland Trust, accessed April 26, 2023, https://www.woodlandtrust.org.uk/visiting-woods/things-to-do/foraging/foraging-guidelines.

189. 'Organoleptic', Oxford English Dictionary, accessed July 25, 2023, https://www.dictionary.com/browse/organoleptic.

190. 'Calendula,' Herbal Reality, February 9, 2023, https://www.herbalreality.com/herb/calendula/.

191. Disha Arora, Anita Rani, and Anupam Sharma, 'A Review on Phytochemistry and Ethnopharmacological Aspects of Genus Calendula,' Pharmacognosy Reviews 7, no. 14 (2013): 179, https://doi.org/10.4103/0973-7847.120520.

192. 'Calendula,' Herbal Reality, February 9, 2023, https://www.herbalreality.com/herb/calendula/.

193. Alieh Kianitalaei et al., 'Althaea Officinalis in Traditional Medicine and Modern Phytotherapy,' Journal of Advanced Pharmacy Education & Research,

2, 9 (2019): 154–61, https://japer.in/storage/models/article/f5TqIxFdtRizpWUR7QJcIhbRLMXjYU2hTii7woeWds9ikCBkEPOjkXbppPnl/althaea-officinalis-in-traditional-medicine-and-modern-phytotherapy.pdf.

194. Shahid Akbar, 'Althaea Officinalis L. (Malvaceae),' essay, in *Handbook of 200 Medicinal Plants* (Springer, 2020), 235–41, https://link.springer.com/chapter/10.1007/978-3-030-16807-0_22#citeas.

195. Alexandra Deters et al., 'Aqueous Extracts and Polysaccharides from Marshmallow Roots (Althea Officinalis L.): Cellular Internalisation and Stimulation of Cell Physiology of Human Epithelial Cells in Vitro,' *Journal of Ethnopharmacology* 127, no. 1 (January 8, 2010): 62–69, https://doi.org/10.1016/j.jep.2009.09.050.

196. Alieh Kianitalaei et al., 'Althaea Officinalis in Traditional Medicine and Modern Phytotherapy,' *Journal of Advanced Pharmacy Education & Research* 2, 9 (2019): 154–61, https://japer.in/storage/models/article/f5TqIxFdtRizpWUR7QJcIhbRLMXjYU2hTii7woeWds9ikCBkEPOjkXbppPnl/althaea-officinalis-in-traditional-medicine-and-modern-phytotherapy.pdf.

197. Sajah Popham, 'Marshmallow: The Great Moistener,' The School of Evolutionary Herbalism, July 4, 2023, https://www.evolutionaryherbalism.com/2022/09/07/marshmallow-the-great-moistener/.

198. 'Forms of Ceremonial and Ritualistic Objects According to Their Functions,' Encyclopædia Britannica, accessed August 3, 2023, https://www.britannica.com/topic/ceremonial-object/Forms-of-ceremonial-and-ritualistic-objects-according-to-their-functions.

199. Arieh Moussaieff et al., 'Incensole Acetate, an Incense Component, Elicits Psychoactivity by Activating TRPV3 Channels in the Brain,' *The FASEB Journal* 22, no. 8 (2008): 3024–34, https://doi.org/10.1096/fj.07-101865.

200. Peter Damian and Kate Damian, *Aromatherapy: Scent and Psyche* (Rochester, Vermont: Healing Arts Press, 1995), 191.

201. 'Boswellia,' IUCN Red List of Threatened Species, accessed August 3, 2023, https://www.iucnredlist.org/search?query=boswellia&searchType=species.

202. Mandy Aftel, *Essence and Alchemy: A Natural History of Perfume* (Layton, UT: Gibbs Smith, 2008), 193.

203. Jennifer Peace Rhind and Stella Hargraves, 'Meditations on Scent,' Sawyer Seminar Series (lecture, Institute for Advanced Studies in the Humanities (IASH), The University of Edinburgh., March 2011), https://www.sensorystudies.org/sensational-investigations/meditations-on-scent/.

204. Jennifer Peace Rhind, *Listening to Scent: An Olfactory Journey with Aromatic Plants and Their Extracts* (London: Singing Dragon, 2014), 41.

205. Tricia Hersey, 'Rest Is Resistance,' The Nap Ministry, January 25, 2023, https://thenapministry.com/.

206. Heidi Borst, 'Epsom Salt: Benefits, Uses and More,' *Forbes*, June 6, 2023, https://www.forbes.com/health/body/epsom-salt/.

207. Mark Moss and Lorraine Oliver, 'Plasma 1,8-Cineole Correlates with Cognitive Performance Following Exposure to Rosemary Essential Oil Aroma,' *Therapeutic Advances in Psychopharmacology* 2, no. 3 (2012): 103–13, https://doi.org/10.1177/2045125312436573.

208. Gabriel Mojay, *Aromatherapy for Healing the Spirit: A Guide to Restoring Emotional and Mental Balance through Essential Oils* (London: Gaia Books Limited, 1999), 115.

209. Peter Damian and Kate Damian, *Aromatherapy: Scent and Psyche* (Rochester, Vermont: Healing Arts Press, 1995), 202.

210. Sawssan Maksoud et al., 'Citrus Aurantium L. Active Constituents, Biological Effects and Extraction Methods. an Updated Review,' *Molecules* 26, no. 19 (2021): 5832, https://doi.org/10.3390/molecules26195832.

211. Carole Fisher, *Materia Medica of Western Herbs* (London, Greater London: Aeon, 2018), 431.

212. Ibid., 246.

213. Ibid., 387.

214. Chopin, Kate, *The Awakening*. (United States: H. S. Stone, 1899). https://archive.org/details/awakeningchop/

215. Süskind, Patrick, *Perfume: The Story of a Murderer* (Penguin Books Limited, 2015. First published 1985).

216. 'Botulism,' NHS choices (NHS, October 3, 2022), https://www.nhs.uk/conditions/botulism/.

INDEX

143

A DAVID AND CHARLES BOOK
© David and Charles, Ltd 2024

David and Charles is an imprint of David and Charles, Ltd, Suite A, Tourism House,
Pynes Hill, Exeter, EX2 5WS

Text © Ellen Rowland 2024
Layout and Illustration © David and Charles, Ltd 2024

First published in the UK and USA in 2024

A catalogue record for this book is available from the British Library.

ISBN-13: 9781446310595 paperback
ISBN-13: 9781446311974 EPUB

This book has been printed on paper from approved suppliers and made from pulp
from sustainable sources.

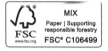

Printed in Turkey by Omur for:
David and Charles, Ltd, Suite A, Tourism House, Pynes Hill, Exeter, EX2 5WS

10 9 8 7 6 5 4 3 2 1

Publishing Director: Ame Verso
Senior Commissioning Editor: Lizzie Kaye
Managing Editor: Jeni Chown
Editor: Jessica Cropper
Project Editor: Jane Trollope
Head of Design: Anna Wade
Design and Illustration: Prudence Rogers
Pre-press Designer: Susan Reansbury
Art Direction: Sarah Rowntree
Photography: Jason Jenkins
Production Manager: Beverley Richardson

David and Charles publishes high-quality books on a wide range of subjects.
For more information visit www.davidandcharles.com.

Follow us on Instagram by searching for @dandcbooks_wellbeing.

Layout of the digital edition of this book may vary depending on reader hardware
and display settings.